The Infant Motor Profile

The Infant Motor Profile is a practical manual on a new, evidence-based method to assess infant motor behaviour.

Not only looking at what milestones the infant has reached, but also paying attention to the quality of motor behaviour – how the infant moves – this text provides professionals involved in the care of infants at risk of developmental disorders with information on five domains of motor behaviour: variation, adaptability, symmetry, fluency, and performance. Backed up by extensive, up-to-date research, it includes percentile curves so that professionals can easily interpret the infants' scores. The profile created from the assessment informs about the infant's current condition and their risk of developmental disorders, as well as providing suggestions for early intervention, tailored to the strengths and limitations of the infant. Used over time, it can be an excellent instrument to monitor the infant's developmental progress.

Illustrated with numerous figures and accompanied by a website hosting over 100 video clips, this text is an essential read for professionals in developmental paediatrics, including paediatric physiotherapists, occupational therapists, developmental paediatricians, neuropaediatricians, and paediatric physiatrists.

Mijna Hadders-Algra is Professor of Developmental Neurology at the Institute for Developmental Neurology, University Medical Center Groningen, The Netherlands.

Kirsten R. Heineman is a practising paediatric neurologist as well as a post-doctoral researcher at the Institute for Developmental Neurology, University Medical Center Groningen, The Netherlands.

The Infant Motor Profile

Mijna Hadders-Algra and
Kirsten R. Heineman

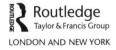
Routledge
Taylor & Francis Group

LONDON AND NEW YORK

First published 2021
by Routledge
2 Park Square, Milton Park, Abingdon, Oxon OX14 4RN

and by Routledge
52 Vanderbilt Avenue, New York, NY 10017

Routledge is an imprint of the Taylor & Francis Group, an informa business

British Library Cataloguing-in-Publication Data
A catalogue record for this book is available from the British Library

Library of Congress Cataloging-in-Publication Data
Names: Hadders-Algra, Mijna, author. | Heineman, Kirsten R., author.
Title: The infant motor profile / Mijna Hadders-Algra and Kirsten R. Heineman.
Description: Milton Park, Abingdon, Oxon ; New York, NY : Routledge, 2021. |
    Includes bibliographical references and index.
Identifiers: LCCN 2020041171 (print) | LCCN 2020041172 (ebook) |
    ISBN 9780367358129 (hardback) | ISBN 9780367358112 (paperback) |
    ISBN 9780429341915 (ebook)
Subjects: LCSH: Motor ability in infants. | Developmental disabilities—
    Risk factors.
Classification: LCC RJ133 .H33 2021 (print) | LCC RJ133 (ebook) |
    DDC 155.4/123—dc23
LC record available at https://lccn.loc.gov/2020041171
LC ebook record available at https://lccn.loc.gov/2020041172

ISBN: 978-0-367-35812-9 (hbk)
ISBN: 978-0-367-35811-2 (pbk)
ISBN: 978-0-429-34191-5 (ebk)

Typeset in Bembo
by Apex CoVantage, LLC

Visit the companion website: www.routledge.com/cw/hadders-algra

Contents

List of figures   vi
List of tables   x
List of boxes   xi
List of videos   xii
Acknowledgements   xiv

1 Introduction   1

2 Principles of neuromotor development   4

3 Design, performance, and psychometric properties of the IMP   17

4 Assessment of motor behaviour while supine   28

5 Assessment of motor behaviour while prone   54

6 Assessment of motor behaviour in the sitting position   72

7 Assessment of motor behaviour while standing and walking   90

8 Assessment of reaching, grasping, and manipulation of objects while sitting   114

9 General: items observed throughout the assessment   128

10 Clinical application and significance of the IMP   132

References   146
Index   155

Figures

2.1   Schematic overview of the developmental processes occurring in
the human brain   5

2.2   Developing human cerebral cortex   6

2.3   Development of primary and secondary variability   12

3.1   Recommended material for the IMP assessment   22

3.2   First page of the IMP-score form   23

4.1   Assessment in supine: starting situation   29

4.2   Objects used to assess reaching, grasping, and manipulation while supine   30

4.3   Assessment of reaching, grasping, and manipulation while supine   31

4.4   Development of the control of head movements while supine in the
norm population (item 1)   32

4.5   Development of adaptability of head movements in the norm
population (item 3)   34

4.6   Development of asymmetry in head position while supine in the
norm population (item 4)   35

4.7   Frequently occurring ATNR on the left side in a three-month-old
infant (item 5)   36

4.8   Hyperextension of neck and trunk in a three-month-old infant (item 6)   37

4.9   Development of manipulative behaviour of hands and fingers in the
norm population (item 7)   38

4.10   Spontaneous movements while supine of two four-month-old infants:
quality of arm and finger movements (items 8 and 9)   39

4.11   Various degrees of tilting of the pelvis (item 10)   41

4.12   Development of tilting of the pelvis in the norm population
(item 10)   42

4.13   Spontaneous movements while supine of two three-month-old infants:
quality of leg and toe movements (items 11 and 12)   43

4.14   Development of rolling from supine into prone in the norm
population (item 13)   45

4.15   Development of reaching, grasping, and manipulation while supine in
the norm population (item 14)   48

4.16   Variation in arm and hand movements during reaching, grasping, and
manipulation while supine (items 16 and 18)   50

4.17   Development of adaptability of arm movements during reaching in
the norm population (item 17)   51

5.1   Starting position while prone in young infants: both shoulders are
       placed in adduction and both elbows in flexion with the hands
       approximately in line with the ears   55
5.2   Head lift while prone in a six-month-old girl: she is able to lift the head
       more than ten seconds and easily turns the head in any direction
       (item 22)   57
5.3   Development of head lift while prone in the norm population (item 22)   57
5.4   Infant of three months with strongly prevailing head position to the left
       while prone; the infant is not able to move the head across the midline
       (item 23)   58
5.5   Asymmetry in head position while prone in the norm population
       (item 23)   59
5.6   Development of adaptability of head movements while prone in the
       norm population (item 25)   60
5.7   Functional ability of shoulder girdle while prone   62
5.8   Development of the functional ability of the shoulder girdle while prone
       in the norm population (item 26)   62
5.9   Functional ability of arms and hands while prone (item 27)   64
5.10   Development of the functional ability of arms and hands while prone in
       the norm population (item 27)   64
5.11   Progression while prone (item 29)   66
5.12   Development of progression while prone, i.e., development of crawling
       in the norm population (item 29)   67
5.13   Infant of five months rolls over the left side from prone into supine
       position (item 31)   69
5.14   Development of rolling from prone into supine in the norm population
       (item 31)   69
5.15   Development of adaptability of crawling in the norm population
       (item 33)   71
6.1   Control of head movements (item 34)   74
6.2   Development of control of head movements while sitting in the norm
       population (item 34)   74
6.3   Development of asymmetry in head position while sitting in the norm
       population (item 35)   75
6.4   Sitting ability (item 36)   77
6.5   Development of sitting ability in the norm population (item 36)   77
6.6   Posture of trunk during independent sitting (item 37)   78
6.7   Development of trunk posture during independent sitting in the norm
       population (item 37)   79
6.8   Development of voluntary arm use during independent sitting in the
       norm population (item 40)   81
6.9   Insufficient variation in sitting movements in an infant of seven months
       (item 41)   82
6.10   Sufficient variation in sitting movements in an infant of 12 months
       (item 41)   83
6.11   Development of adaptability of sitting movements in the norm
       population (item 42)   84

6.12   Various ways to get into a sitting position (item 43)   85
6.13   Infant of eight months in a half-sitting position; this performance does
       not credit for score 2 at item 43   86
6.14   Development of getting into a sitting position in the norm population
       (item 43)   86
6.15   Development of adaptability of getting into a sitting position in the
       norm population (item 45)   88
6.16   The infant moves forward by means of bottom shuffling (item 46)   89
7.1   Standing ability (item 47)   92
7.2   Development of standing ability in the norm population (item 47)   92
7.3   Standing up (item 48)   94
7.4   Development of standing up in the norm population (item 48)   94
7.5   Infant of 12 months with sufficient variation in standing up movements
       (item 49)   95
7.6   Development of adaptability of standing up in the norm population
       (item 50)   97
7.7   Infant of 12 months who just mastered independent walking (item 51)   98
7.8   Development of walking in the norm population (item 51)   98
7.9   Development of balance during independent walking in the norm
       population (item 52)   100
7.10   High guard arm posture during independent walking in an infant
       aged 13 months (item 53)   101
7.11   Development of arm posture and movements during independent
       walking in the norm population (item 53)   102
7.12   Development of adaptability of the movements of arms and hands during
       independent walking in the norm population (item 56)   105
7.13   Development of adaptability of trunk movements while standing and
       independent walking in the norm population (item 58)   107
7.14   Development of adaptability of leg movements during independent
       walking in the norm population (item 61)   109
7.15   Development of heel-toe gait during independent walking in the norm
       population (item 62)   110
7.16   Development of adaptability of feet movements during independent
       walking in the norm population (item 64)   112
8.1   Evaluation of reaching, grasping, and manipulation while sitting on the
       caregiver's lap   115
8.2   Infant of 14 months being able to reach towards and hold at least three
       objects (item 66)   117
8.3   Development of reaching, grasping, and manipulation of objects in a
       sitting position in the norm population (item 66)   118
8.4   Variation in arm and hand movements during reaching, grasping, and
       manipulation in a sitting position (items 68 and 71)   120
8.5   Development of adaptability of reaching movements of the arm in a
       sitting position in the norm population (item 69)   121
8.6   Type of grasping (item 70)   123
8.7   Development of the type of grasping in the norm population (item 70)   123

8.8 Development of adaptability of hand movements during reaching, grasping, and manipulation in a sitting position in the norm population (item 72)   125
9.1 Variation in facial expression (item 75)   128
9.2 Marked drooling reflected by the large wet spot on the infant's clothes (item 77)   129
10.1 Percentile curves of the IMP adaptability domain in 1100 infants aged 7–17 months   135
10.2 Percentile curves of the IMP performance domain in 1700 infants aged 2–18 months   139
10.3 Percentile curves of the total IMP scores in 1700 infants aged 2–18 months   141

Tables

3.1   Recommendations on the practical procedures of the IMP   20
3.2   Background characteristics of children participating in the IMP
       norm study (n=1,700)   24
3.3   Associations between perinatal and socio-economic factors and
       low IMP scores in the IMP-SINDA norm population,
       logistic regression analyses, n=1,600 infants   26
3.4   Concurrent validity of IMP and SINDA: associations between low
       IMP scores (<5th percentile) and atypical SINDA neurological score
       in the IMP-SINDA norm population (odds ratio and confidence
       interval)   26
10.1 Percentile values for the scores of the IMP variation, symmetry, and
       fluency domains   134
10.2 Age-dependent percentile values for the adaptability domain scores 136
10.3 Age-dependent percentile values for the performance domain scores   140
10.4 Age-dependent percentile values of the total IMP scores   142
10.5 Percentile ranks of the total IMP score by age (in months)   142
10.6 IMP profile and suggestions for intervention   143

Boxes

1.1   Two examples of application of the IMP in clinical practice   2
3.1   Calculation of the IMP scores – background details   18
10.1 Computation of IMP percentile curves   132
10.2 The two clinical examples in Chapter 1   144

Videos

Accompanying videos can be accessed on the book's companion website at www.routledge.com/cw/hadders-algra

4.1 Assessment in supine position
4.2 Assessment of head movements in supine
4.3 Variation and adaptability of head movements in supine (items 2 and 3)
4.4 Strongly prevailing head position in supine (item 4)
4.5 Manipulative behaviour of fingers in supine (item 7)
4.6 Variation in arm and finger movements in supine (items 8 and 9)
4.7 Variation in leg and toe movements in supine (items 11 and 12)
4.8 Rolling from supine into prone (item 13)
4.9 Reaching, grasping and manipulation in supine (item 14)
4.10 Reaching, grasping and manipulation in supine, presence of asymmetry (item 15)
4.11 Variation in arm and hand movements during reaching and grasping in supine (items 16 and 18)
4.12 Adaptability of arm and hand movements during reachging, grasping and manipulation in supine (items 17 and 19)
4.13 Tremor during reaching and grasping (item 20)
4.14 Fluency of movements in supine (item 21)
5.1 Assessment in prone
5.2 Head lift in prone (item 22)
5.3 Prevailing head position in prone (item 23)
5.4 Adaptability of head movements in prone (item 25)
5.5 Functional ability of shoulder girdle in prone (item 26)
5.6 Functional ability of arms and hands in prone (item 27)
5.7 Posture and movements of arms and hands during activity in prone, presence of asymmetry (item 28)
5.8 Progression in prone: development of crawling (item 29)
5.9 Variation in pre-crawling movements of the legs (item 30)
5.10 Variation in crawling (item 32)
5.11 Adaptability of crawling (item 33)
6.1 Assessment in sitting position
6.2 Prevailing head position in sitting (item 34)
6.3 Sitting ability (item 36)
6.4 Posture of trunk and legs during sitting, asymmetries (item 38)
6.5 Posture and movements of arms and hands during sitting or supported sitting, presence of asymmetry (item 39)

6.6   Uses arms for voluntary activities (item 40)
6.7   Variation and adaptability in sitting movements (item 41)
6.8   Variation in getting into sitting position (item 44)
6.9   Adaptability of getting into sitting position (item 45)
6.10 Bottom shuffling (item 46)
7.1   Assessment of standing and walking
7.2   Standing ability (item 47)
7.3   Standing up (item 48)
7.4   Variation in standing up behaviour (item 49)
7.5   Adaptability of standing up behaviour (item 50)
7.6   Walking (item 51)
7.7   Balance during walking (item 52)
7.8   Arm posture and movements during walking (item 53)
7.9   Asymmetry of arm posture and movements during independent walking (item 54)
7.10 Variation in movements of arms and hands during independent walking (item 55)
7.11 Variation of trunk, legs and feet postures and movements during standing and independent walking (items 57, 60 and 63)
7.12 Adaptability of trunk, legs and feet postures and movements during standing and independent walking (items 58, 61 and 64)
7.13 Asymmetry in leg movements during standing and walking (item 59)
7.14 Heel-toe gait during independent walking (item 62)
7.15 Fluency of movements during independent walking (item 65)
8.1   Reaching, grasping and manipulation of objects in sitting (item 66)
8.2   Reaching, grasping and manipulation, asymmetry (item 67)
8.3   Variation and adaptability in reaching movements of the arms during sitting (items 68 and 69)
8.4   Variation and adaptability of hand movements during reaching, grasping and manipulation in sitting (items 71 and 72)
8.5   Tremor and non-fluent movements during reaching in sitting (items 73 and 74)
9.1   Stereotyped tongue movements (item 78)

Acknowledgements

The work described in this book is the result of the collaboration and contribution of many people. We are especially grateful for the wonderful and skilled assistance of Anneke Kracht, who produced all figures and video clips. We also wish to express our great thanks for the statistical support of Dr. Sacha la Bastide-van Gemert, who calculated the IMP percentile curves.

The collection of the Dutch norm data would not have been possible without the contribution of the colleagues of the KinderAcademie in Groningen (heads: Selma de Ruiter, PhD, and Francien Geerds, MSc), of many medical master students from the University of Groningen, and of Ying-Chin Wu, PT, PhD, and Patricia van Iersel, PT, PhD. Last but not least, we thank the many parents and infants who participated in the studies underlying the IMP manual, in particular those who allowed us to use images (figures and/or videoclips) of their infants to illustrate the IMP.

The collection of the norm data was part of the IMP-SINDA project that was financially supported by the CorneliaStichting and the Stichting Ontwikkelingsneurofysiologie Groningen. We also acknowledge the technical assistance of Linze Dijkstra in the IMP-SINDA project and the critical and constructive comments of Schirin Akhbari Ziegler PT, PhD, on drafts of some of the chapters.

Mijna Hadders-Algra and Kirsten R. Heineman

1 Introduction

Developmental disorders are disorders originating from the disruption of developmental processes during foetal and early postnatal life, due to a mix of genetic, social, prenatal, perinatal, and neonatal risk factors (Hadders-Algra 2018a). Examples are cerebral palsy (CP), developmental coordination disorder (DCD), and autism spectrum disorders. Accumulating evidence indicates that infants at high risk of or with developmental disorders may profit from early intervention (Spittle et al. 2015, Morgan et al. 2016, Hadders-Algra et al. 2017): that is, intervention at an age when the brain is characterized by high plasticity. This invokes the need for early detection of these infants.

Early detection is based on clinical history (e.g., preterm birth, intrauterine growth retardation, hypoxic-ischaemic encephalopathy, a complex congenital heart disease), early neuroimaging (in particular, magnetic resonance imaging [MRI] or cranial ultrasound scans), and a neurodevelopmental assessment of the infant (Novak et al. 2017). The neurodevelopmental assessment that predicts the development of outcome best is the General Movement Assessment (Einspieler et al. 2005, Heineman and Hadders-Algra 2008, Bosanquet et al. 2013). However, because general movements disappear between three and five months corrected age (CA), it is not possible to use this assessment in older infants. This inspired us to develop the Infant Motor Profile (IMP) (Heineman and Hadders-Algra 2008, Heineman et al. 2008).

The IMP is – like the General Movement Assessment – based on a video evaluation of the quality of spontaneous motor behaviour. Quintessential to General Movement Assessment is the evaluation of movement complexity and variation, which may be regarded as the spatial and temporal components of movement variation (Hadders-Algra 2018b, Wu et al. 2020c). It evaluates the size of the infant's movement repertoire (Hadders-Algra 2021b). In addition, General Movement Assessment evaluates the presence of age-specific movement characteristics, especially the presence of fidgety movements at two to five months CA (Einspieler et al. 2005, Wu et al. 2020a).

Variation is a hallmark of neural activity and typical motor development (Touwen 1976, Edelman 1989, Changeux 1997, Chervyakov et al. 2016). This stimulated Gerald Edelman (1989, 1993) to develop the Neuronal Group Selection Theory (NGST) (for details see Chapter 2). The concepts of the NGST have been used to develop the IMP, in particular to design its two novel motor domains: variation (the size of the movement repertoire) and adaptability (the ability to select from the motor repertoire the strategy that suits the situation best) (Heineman et al. 2008, Hadders-Algra 2010, 2018c). In addition to these two new domains, the IMP contains three traditional domains that describe movement symmetry, fluency, and motor performance.

The IMP is a method designed to evaluate the motor behaviour of infants aged 3 to 18 months CA. However, in infants with developmental disorders or developmental delays, the IMP may also be applied after the age of 18 months, up to the age when the child has managed to walk independently for a couple of months. The IMP is based on a video recording of a semi-standardized play session of about 15 minutes, during which an assessor plays with the infant in such a way that the IMP items can be assessed. This means that the playing assessor has knowledge of the IMP items, allowing her to adapt the assessment to the infant's functional abilities and the IMP needs. The 80 items of the IMP evaluate motor behaviour in supine and prone positions; while sitting, standing, and walking; when reaching and grasping; and during manipulation. It is a discriminative, evaluative, and predictive measurement. The IMP has been developed for health care professionals working in the field of early detection of developmental disorders and early intervention: for instance, paediatric physiotherapists, paediatric occupational therapists, neuropaediatricians, and developmental paediatricians (see Box 1.1).

Box 1.1   Two examples of application of the IMP in clinical practice

Example 1: James

A paediatric physiotherapist is seeing James, a boy referred because of positional head preference to the right side. James's prenatal and perinatal history had been uneventful. The therapist performs an IMP assessment when James is three months old. The IMP shows low scores in the domains of variation and symmetry (both below the 5th percentile [<P5]), the score on fluency is within the typical range, and the performance score is below the 15th percentile (<P15). The therapist guides James and his family, stressing the need for varied motor experiences and explicit stimulation of James's non-preferred left side. After three months, the therapist repeats the IMP assessment. The results show that James has improved in the performance domain (P15–P50), but the symmetry score improved to a limited extent only (still <P5), and the variation score remains low (<P5). The therapist considers the latter especially as a sign of a high risk of a developmental disorder. She refers James and his family to a paediatric neurologist.

Example 2: Janet

A paediatrician is in charge of the follow-up of a preterm girl, Janet. She was born at 27 weeks of gestation and had a complicated neonatal history, and the MRI scan of her brain showed mild periventricular white matter abnormalities. The paediatrician assesses Janet at eight months corrected age with the IMP. She notices the following: (1) Janet's variation score is relatively good (a score just below the 50th percentile [P15–P50]), suggesting that Janet's risk of CP is low, which carries a reassuring message for the parents; (2) the symmetry and fluency scores are within the typical range; and (3) Janet's adaptability and performance scores are below the 15th percentile (<P15). The latter two scores imply that the infant may profit from early intervention: that is, the type of intervention in which caregivers learn how they can stimulate the infant's development best (Hadders-Algra 2021a).

These example cases will be picked up again in Chapter 10.

The infant's self-generated activity is crucial in the IMP. The self-produced motor actions – generated entirely spontaneously or as part of the IMP play with the assessor – are scored according to the defined criteria of 80 items. The IMP evaluation is based on observation of motor behaviour and does not involve interpretations of motor behaviour (e.g., 'high muscle tone'). Interpretation of the IMP data occurs on the basis of the IMP domain scores and the IMP total score, which are calculated at the end of the assessment (see Chapter 10). The observational nature of the IMP is in line with the ethological approach of Heinz Prechtl, the pioneer of General Movement Assessment (Prechtl 1990). Prechtl learned the value of ethological methods, including behavioural observation, from his famous teacher, the Nobel laureate Konrad Lorenz.

Chapter 2 summarizes the principles of neuromotor development and pays special attention to the NGST. Chapter 3 describes the design of the IMP and its psychometric properties. It also pays attention to the practicalities of the assessment. Chapters 4 to 9 report the actual assessment procedures for the different situations during which the motor behaviour is evaluated (supine, prone, sitting, standing and walking, reaching, grasping, and manipulation). The individual items are described, including the criteria for their scores. For the items with age dependencies, the dependence on the infant's age is illustrated with graphs from our norm data study (see Chapter 3). Dependence predominantly occurs in the items of the domains performance and adaptability.

In Chapter 10, the calculation and interpretation of the IMP scores are discussed. This chapter includes percentile curves based on the data of our norms data study of a representative sample of 1,700 infants of the Netherlands, aged 2 to 18 months CA. The percentile curves assist the interpretation of the IMP scores. We describe the significance of the IMP profile for the infant's actual physiotherapeutic guidance and the significance of the IMP for prediction of developmental outcome.

Finally, three practical remarks: first, the infant ages used in this manual always refer to ages corrected for preterm birth. This is not further indicated in the text.

Second, writing about individuals who may belong to any gender category puts an author in the awkward position of either using complex expressions or the selection of a specific gender. The latter results in a text which is easier to read, but this option has the disadvantage that an impression of 'neglect' of other gender identities may occur. We opted for the single gender option to facilitate readability and chose the female gender when referring to the examiner and the male gender when referring to the child. However, we would like to stress our gender-neutral intentions.

Third, the book is richly illustrated, both with figures and videos. The parents of the infants all gave written permission for us to use the video and photo material for publication. In the remaining chapters, this information is not repeated at each figure or video.

2 Principles of neuromotor development

The IMP is an instrument for the evaluation of motor behaviour in the age range of 3 to 18 months. During this period of life, the infant's motor behaviour changes impressively: for instance, typically developing infants learn to reach and grasp and to sit, stand, and walk. Infants acquire these skills due to a continuous interaction between developmental processes occurring in the body and the environment. Of the developmental changes to the body, those occurring in the brain play a prominent role. In this chapter, we briefly summarize (1) human brain development, (2) muscle development, (3) development of the sensory systems, (4) theories of motor development, and (5) motor development. Our focus is on the developmental changes occurring before the age of two years (Hadders-Algra 2021a). In the section on the theories of motor development, we zoom in on the Neuronal Group Selection Theory, as it is the theoretical framework underlying the IMP.

Human brain development

The development of the human brain takes many years; it is not until the age of 40 that the nervous system obtains its full-blown adult configuration (De Graaf-Peters and Hadders-Algra 2006, Hadders-Algra 2018a; Figure 2.1). The developmental processes in the brain are the result of a continuous interaction between genes and environment, activity and experience (Ben-Ari and Spitzer 2010).

Neural development starts in the fifth week postmenstrual age (PMA) with the ectodermal development of the neural tube. Shortly after tube closure, specific areas near the ventricles start to generate neurons. The majority of neurons are formed between 5 and 25 to 28 weeks PMA. From their origin in the ventricular layers, the neurons move radially or tangentially to their final place of destination in the more superficially located cortical plate (Ortega et al. 2018). The process of migration peaks between 20 and 26 weeks PMA. During migration, the neurons start to differentiate: that is, they start to produce axons, dendrites, synapses with neurotransmitters, the intracellular machinery, and the complex neuronal membranes. Remarkably, the first generation of neurons does not migrate to the cortical plate; they halt in the cortical subplate.

The cortical subplate is a structure between the cortical plate and the future white matter (Figure 2.2). It is the major site of neuronal differentiation and synaptogenesis in the cortex, it receives the first ingrowing cortical afferents (e.g., from the thalamus), and it is the main site of synaptic activity in the mid-foetal brain (Kostović et al. 2015). This implies that the subplate is a major mediator of foetal motor behaviour (Hadders-Algra 2018b). The subplate is thickest between 28 and 34 weeks PMA. Before that age, from

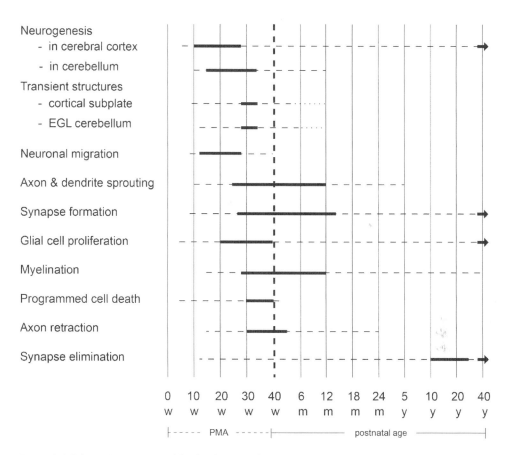

Figure 2.1 Schematic overview of the developmental processes occurring in the human brain. The bold lines indicate that the processes mentioned on the left are very active; the broken lines denote that the processes still continue, but less abundantly. The diagram is based on the review of Hadders-Algra (2018a).

EGL = external granular layer; m = months; PMA = postmenstrual age; w = weeks; y = years.

Figure reproduced with permission from *Early Detection and Early Intervention in Developmental Motor Disorders* by Mijna Hadders-Algra (ed) published by Mac Keith Press (www.mackeith.co.uk) in its Clinics in Developmental Medicine Series, 2021, 978-1-911612-43-8.

25 to 26 weeks onwards, subplate neurons start to die off gradually, and later-generated neurons begin to populate the cortical plate. These developmental changes are accompanied by a relocation of the thalamocortical afferents, which now grow to their final target in the cortical plate (Kostović et al. 2014a).

In the third trimester of gestation, the cortex increases in size, and gyrification starts (Kostović and Judas 2010). During this phase, the thickness of the subplate decreases, while the cortical plate increases. This also implies that the human cortex at this time is characterized by the co-existence of two separate but interconnected cortical circuitries: the transient foetal circuitries centred in the subplate and the immature, but progressively

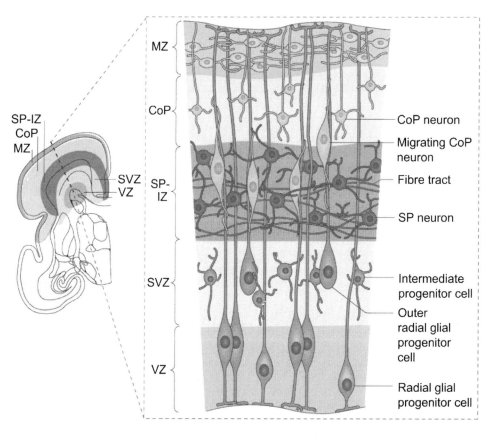

Figure 2.2 Developing human cerebral cortex. Schematic representation of the human cerebral cortex at 28 weeks PMA. On the left a coronal section is shown; the inset box on the right provides details of the developmental processes. The ventricular zone (VZ) and subventricular zone (SVZ) constitute the germinal matrices where cell division occurs. The first generations of cells are generated in the VZ, the later generations in the SVZ. The SVZ is a structure that expanded during phylogeny; it is especially large in primates (Ortega et al. 2018). The radial glial cells span their shafts between between the germinal layers and the outer layer of the cortex (marginal zone (MZ)). The first generation neurons have migrated to the subplate (SP) – they participate in the functional fetal cortex; later generations of neurons migrate to the cortical plate (CP).

Figure reproduced from Hoerder-Suabedissen and Molnár (2015) with permission from the authors and the Nature Publishing Group.

developing, permanent circuitry centred in the cortical plate. The double circuitry state ends when the subplate has dissolved. This situation is reached in the primary motor, sensory, and visual cortices around three months post-term, but first around the age of one year in the associative prefrontal cortex (Kostović et al. 2014b).

Brain development also involves the creation of glial cells. Glial cell production occurs in the second half of gestation in particular. Part of the glial cells (i.e., the oligodendrocytes) take care of axonal myelination. Oligodendrocyte development peaks between 28 and 40 weeks PMA (Volpe 2009a). Myelination is prominently present in the third trimester of gestation and the first six months postnatally (Yakovlev and Lecours 1967, Haynes et al. 2005). However, myelination is a long-lasting process that is first completed around the age of 40 years (De Graaf-Peters and Hadders-Algra 2006).

Brain development does not only imply the generation of neurons and connections; it also involves regressive phenomena. The process of neuronal death has already been mentioned. It is estimated that in the mammalian central nervous system, about half the created neurons die off through apoptosis. The neurons die as the result of inter-action between endogenously programmed processes and chemical and electrical sig-nals induced by experience (Lossi and Merighi 2003). A well-known example of axon elimination is the removal occurring during corticospinal tract development. In this tract, axon elimination starts during the last trimester of gestation and continues during the first two postnatal years. As a result, the tract's initially bilateral corticospinal projections in the spinal cord are reorganized into a mainly contralateral fibre system (Eyre 2007). The elimination of synapses in the brain starts during the mid-foetal period. However, in the cerebral cortex synapse, elimination is most pronounced between the onset of puberty and early adulthood (Petanjek et al. 2011).

From early age onwards, neurotransmitters and their receptors are present in neural tissue. (For a review, see Herlenius and Lagercrantz [2010].) Interestingly, the peri-term period is characterized by a transient specific setting of various transmitter systems: that is, by a temporary overexpression of the noradrenergic α2-receptors and glutamatergic NMDA-receptors, a relatively high serotonergic innervation, and a high dopaminer-gic turnover. It has been suggested that this neurotransmitter setting around term age induces an increased excitability, expressed, amongst other ways, by the motoneurons, and that this temporary transmitter setting facilitates the transition from the foetal periodic breathing pattern to the continuous breathing needed for postnatal survival (Hadders-Algra 2018b).

The development of the cerebellum has its own timing. Cells in the cerebellum originate from two proliferative zones: (1) the ventricular zone which brings forth the deep cerebellar nuclei and the Purkinje cells, and (2) the external granular layer origi-nating from the rhombic lip (Volpe 2009b). Cell proliferation in the cerebellum starts at 11 weeks PMA in the ventricular zone and at 15 weeks in the external granular layer. The external granular layer is a transient structure reaching its peak thickness between 28 and 34 weeks PMA. It produces the most numerous cells of the cerebellum, the granule cells. These cells migrate from the external granular layer inward to their final destination in the internal granular layer. The latter grows most prominently between mid-gestation and three months post-term. The external granular layer shrinks, in particular between two and three months post-term. However, it takes until the sec-ond half of the first postnatal year for the external granular layer to dissolve entirely (Hadders-Algra 2018a).

In summary, during foetal life and the first two years post-term, the brain shows high developmental activity. The most significant changes occur in the second half of gestation and the first three months post-term, in particular in the cortical subplate and cerebellum. As the transient subplate pairs a high rate of intricate developmental changes and interac-tions with clear functional activity, two phases of development have been distinguished: (1) the transient cortical subplate phase, ending around three months post-term, when the permanent circuitries in the primary motor, somatosensory, and visual cortices have replaced the temporary ones in the subplate and, subsequently, (2) the phase in which the permanent circuitries dominate. In the latter phase, in particular during the remainder of the first post-term year, the brain's major developmental changes consist of axon recon-figuration, dendrite and synapse production, abundant myelination, and an integration of the permanent circuitries in the association areas (Hadders-Algra 2018a).

Muscle development

Muscle tissue has a mesodermic origin. From five to eight weeks PMA, undifferentiated mesenchymal cells start to produce actin and myosin; when these proteins assemble into filaments, the myoblast is born. Shortly thereafter, adjacent myoblasts fuse into myotubes, which are the most prominent muscle cells between 8 and 16 weeks PMA. Between 16 and 20 weeks PMA, myotubes start to change into myocytes. The myocytes are promi-nent producers of contractile myofilaments and myofibrils (Sarnat 2004).

In the subsequent weeks, especially between 20 and 30 weeks PMA, the histochemi-cal differentiation into type I and type II myocytes (or muscle fibres) starts; this process is under neural control. Type I fibres are characterized by a strong oxidative enzymatic activ-ity and a relatively weak glycolytic activity, implying that they are fatigue resistant. Type II fibres have a relatively weak oxidative and a relatively strong glycolytic enzymatic activity. They are capable of quickly generating a relatively large force output, but they fatigue eas-ily. Around 30 weeks PMA, about half the muscle fibres are characterized as type I and the other half as type II. The type II fibres further specialize into types IIa and IIb, the latter being able to quickly produce high forces at the expense of fast fatiguing. The characteris-tics of type IIa fibres fall between those of type I and type IIb fibres. At term, 15% to 20% of the type II fibres are still classified as undifferentiated (IIc) (Sarnat 2004).

After term age, the number of muscle fibres does not change – it is genetically deter-mined. But, of course, the muscle fibres and therewith the muscles continue to grow, and they gradually obtain their specific muscle characteristics. For instance, the soleus muscle attains its high percentage of fibre I fibres at the age of 9 to 12 months (Sarnat 2004).

Development of sensory systems

Development of the visual system

After birth, visual information is a major source of afferent input used in motor develop-ment. Short visual fixation and some visual following of a target with strong black and white contrasts is present in low-risk preterm infants at 31 to 33 weeks PMA (Ricci et al. 2010). Yet the infant's visual acuity at term is 40-fold less than that of the adult (Miranda 1970). Acuity rapidly improves during the first month, but at one month, the infant's visual acuity still falls short of the adult's by a factor of 12 (Braddick and Atkinson 2011). Around the age of four to six months, the development of visual acuity plateaus for about five months. Thereafter, visual acuity gradually improves. However, it takes about seven to nine years before visual acuity has reached adult values (Adams and Courage 2002).

Two other visual functions are not present at term age: colour vision and stereop-sis. Colour vision emerges at around two months (Burr et al. 1996). At three months, yellow-blue targets are easily detected, but it takes between 17 and 23 months before all infants are able to detect red-green targets (Mercer et al. 2014). The precursor of stere-opsis (binocular summation) also emerges at two months, while stereopsis itself starts at four to five months. However, it takes till early adolescence for stereo-acuity to obtain its adult capacity (Norcia and Gerhard 2015).

Development of the vestibular system

The vestibular system assists human beings in spatial orientation and balance control. Structural development of the labyrinth with its semicircular canals and otoliths (responsible for the detection of angular and linear acceleration, respectively) occurs in large part during the first half of gestation (Jeffery and Spoor 2004). The presence of the vestibular-ocular reflex and the Moro reflex in preterm infants indicates that the vestibular system is functionally active prior to term age (Dubowitz et al. 1999; vestibular-ocular reflex: personal observation).

   Most data on the development of the vestibular system during infancy are based on sparse studies using the vestibular-ocular reflex: that is, the reflexive adaptation of movements of the eyes to the movements of the head on the basis of vestibular information. These studies show that vestibular responsiveness improves quickly during the first two months post-term (Weissman et al. 1989, Young 2015). Next, the vestibular-ocular reflex continues to improve until the age of six years, after which development slowly progresses until the age of 16 years (Wiener-Vacher and Wiener 2017).

Development of proprioception

Proprioception provides the nervous system with information on muscles, tendons, and joints. Studies on monosynaptic stretch reflexes show that these reflexes are present from at least 31 weeks PMA onwards (O'Sullivan et al. 1991). With increasing age, the threshold to elicit the response increases, starting with a relatively rapid increase during the first three months post-term, which is followed by a slow and gradual increase until the age of six years (Hakamada et al. 1988, O'Sullivan et al. 1991). During infancy, the monosynaptic stretch reflex elicits activity not only in its homonymous muscle, but also in other muscles. For instance, after a biceps brachii tendon tap, reflex activity variably irradiates to the triceps, pectoralis major, deltoid, and hypothenar muscles, and during the knee jerk, reflex activity variably irradiates to the ipsilateral hamstrings, gastrocnemius, and tibialis anterior muscles and the contralateral quadriceps and hamstrings muscles (O'Sullivan et al. 1991, Leonard et al. 1995, Teulier et al. 2011, Hamer et al. 2016). With increasing age, reflex irradiation decreases, but in the second year of life, it is still present in many muscles. It disappears at the age of four to five years (O'Sullivan et al. 1991, Leonard et al. 1995). These data indicate that spinal circuitries involved in segmental processing of proprioceptive information show substantial developmental changes, including changes in reciprocal and Renshaw inhibition (McDonough et al. 2001). These changes occur in interdependence with supraspinal developmental changes.

Development of the processing of cutaneous information

Cutaneous input supplies the nervous system with information received by the skin: for example, from painful stimuli, from the skin of body parts in touch with a support surface, or from the hands during manipulation. The development of the processing of cutaneous information at early age has been studied especially by means of the flexion withdrawal reflex (stimulation of the foot sole results in flexion of the stimulated leg). This reflex has been observed in preterm infants from 23 weeks PMA onwards (Martakis et al. 2017). In young preterm infants, the reflex has a very low reflex threshold; its receptive field extends to the thigh and buttock, and it shows sensitization: that is, upon repeated stimulation, a build-up of the response occurs, finally resulting in generalized body movements (Andrews and Fitzgerald 1994). With increasing age, the threshold increases, the size of the response decreases, the receptive field gets smaller, and – between 35 and 37 weeks PMA – sensitization changes to habituation (Andrews and Fitzgerald 1994, Fabrizi et al. 2011, Hartley et al. 2016). These developmental changes are paralleled by changes in evoked responses in the electroencephalogram (EEG). Before 35 to 37 weeks PMA, both a nociceptive stimulus (clinically required heel lance) and a non-nociceptive stimulus (touch) only evoke non-specific bursts in the EEG, but after this age, these stimuli result in distinct evoked responses that differ for the nociceptive and non-nociceptive stimulus (Fabrizi et al. 2011, Hartley et al. 2016). These changes suggest significant changes in the supraspinal circuitries, in which the increasing relocation of the thalamocortical afferents in the cortical plate presumably plays a role.

Full-term neonates already have amazing abilities to process haptic information with their hands: they are able to discriminate objects on the basis of weight (Hernandez-Reif et al. 2001), texture density (Molina and Jouen 2003), and rigidity or elasticity (Rochat 1987). They even show signs of cross-modal recognition of shape: that is, they are able to transfer tactile shape information received by the hands to visual information (Streri and Gentaz 2003).

Knowledge of the processing of cutaneous information stems especially from studies on cutaneomuscular reflexes. A typical cutaneomuscular reflex has three components: E1, a positive response at short spinal latency, which is followed by an inhibitory response (I1), which in turn is followed by E2, the second positive response in which supraspinal circuitries play a significant role. During infancy, E1 is the most prominent feature of the response. From about six months onwards, I1 emerges, whereas E2 appears between one-and-a-half and four years of age (Issler and Stephens 1983, Evans et al. 1990). In children younger than six years, E2 is smaller than E1, whereas in the majority of children older than 12 years, E2 has become larger than E1 (Evans et al. 1990). The data indicate that with increasing age, supraspinal systems play an increasing role in the processing of cutaneous information. The central processing of somatosensory information is getting faster with increasing age, in particular during the first three postnatal years. It obtains adult values at the age of seven to eight years (Lauffer and Wenzel 1986).

Development of the auditory system

Auditory information is not only a primary input source for language development; it also allows for the processing of spoken feedback on motor activities, and it serves spatial orientation. From 19 weeks PMA, the foetus is able to respond to tones with movements. Initially, only responses to low tones occur. At 27 weeks, foetuses respond to tones of 250 and 500 Hz, but not to tones of 1,000 and 3,000 Hz. From 33 to 35 weeks PMA, the higher tones are added to the auditory repertoire. During the second half of gestation, the volume needed to elicit a response decreases by 20 to 30 dB (Hepper and Shahidullah 1994).

At term age, auditory development already allows neonates to distinguish the maternal voice from the voice of a female stranger (Kisilevsky et al. 2003) and to discriminate between native and non-native vowels (Moon et al. 2013). Yet the tone detection threshold of term neonates is 30 to 70 dB higher than that of adults. This threshold rapidly decreases during the first six months post-term, especially for high tones, so that at six months, the threshold for these tones is only 10 dB higher than that in adults. The sensitivity for high tones continues to develop faster than that for low tones, with the former reaching adult values at around two years and the latter at around ten years (Mattock et al. 2012).

Development of the processing of olfactory and gustatory information

The chemical senses of smell and taste primarily serve the evaluation of nutritional substances. But in infants, these senses also assist in the development of motor behaviour, in particular the development of reaching, grasping, and manipulation. Infants do not just explore objects with their hands and eyes. They virtually always combine manual and visual exploration with probing by mouth; the mouthing serves the multimodal exploration of objects (Hadders-Algra 2018c). Mouthing continues to be a favourite means of object exploration during the first nine months post-term but shows a significant decline thereafter (Ruff 1984).

Theories on motor development

Concepts of motor behaviour largely changed during the last century. The earlier view that motor behaviour was primarily organized in chains of reflexes was replaced by the notion that spontaneous, intrinsic activity is a quintessential feature of the brain (Sherrington 1906, Raichle 2015). Concurrently, the ideas on motor development changed. During the major part of the past century, the Neural Maturationist Theories guided developmental thinking (e.g., Gesell and Amatruda 1947). These theories considered motor development basically as an innate, maturational process. But during the last two decades of last century, it became clear that motor development is largely affected by experience. This insight and our limited knowledge of the mechanisms underlying motor development generated a wealth of motor developmental theories.

Currently, two theoretical frameworks are dominant: the Dynamic Systems Theory (Thelen 1995, Smith and Thelen 2003, Spencer et al. 2011) and the Neuronal Group Selection Theory (NGST) (Edelman 1989, 1993, Hadders-Algra 2010, 2018c). These frameworks share the opinion that motor development is a non-linear process with a multifactorial origin and phases of transition. The contributing factors consist of features of the child itself, such as body weight and muscle power; the presence of health problems, such as a cardiac disorder; and components of the environment, such as housing conditions, the composition of the family, and the presence of toys. In other words, both theories acknowledge the importance of experience and context. But the two theories differ in their opinion of the role of genetically determined neurodevelopmental processes. Genetic factors of the make-up of the brain play only a limited role in the Dynamic Systems Theory, whereas in NGST, genetic information, epigenetic cascades, and experience play equally prominent roles in brain and motor development (Edelman 1989, 1993, Hadders-Algra 2010, 2018a). As the latter corresponds better to current insights into the complexities of genetic and epigenetic control of neural development (Kang et al. 2011, Lv et al. 2013), we used the NGST as the reference framework for the design of the IMP.

NGST and typical motor development

NGST's starting point is the variation in neural behaviour (Edelman 1989, 1993, Chervyakov et al. 2016). According to NGST, motor development is characterized by two phases of variability: primary and secondary variability[1] (Edelman 1989). The borders of variability are determined by genetic instructions (Krubitzer and Kaas 2005, Chervyakov et al. 2016). Development starts with the phase of primary variability, during which the spontaneous activity of the nervous system tries out all available functional options (Leighton and Lohmann 2016). In terms of motor behaviour, this means that the nervous system explores all motor possibilities of its repertoires, therewith inducing abundant variation in motor behaviour (Hadders-Algra 2010, 2018c). Varied motor behaviour emerges at nine to ten weeks PMA, implying that the onset of varied motility coincides with the emergence of synaptic activity in the cortical subplate (Figure 2.3; Hadders-Algra 2018b). The varied motor exploration generates a wealth of self-produced afferent information, which in turn is used directly or indirectly via transcriptional gene expression for further sculpting of the nervous system (experience-expectant development) (Greenough et al. 1987). However, initially (i.e., during the phase of primary variability), the afferent information can only be used to a limited extent to adapt motor behaviour

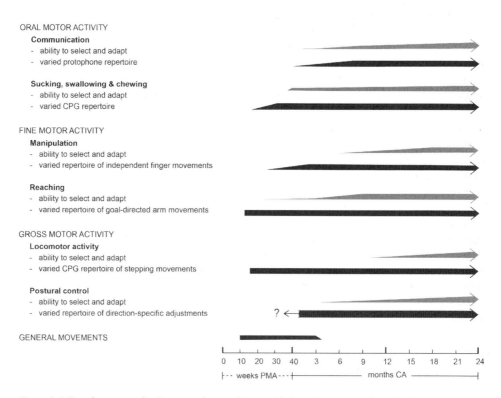

Figure 2.3 Development of primary and secondary variability. Overview of the development of the phases of primary and secondary variability in gross, fine, and oral motor development. The bottom line denotes age, first in weeks PMA, after term (40 weeks) in months corrected age. The black timelines reflect the development of the varied repertoire, the grey timelines that of the ability to select and adapt. The diagram indicates that the primary repertoires primarily develop prior to term age, whereas secondary variability, i.e., the ability to select and adapt, mainly develops after three months post-term. An exception to this rule is the development of adaptive sucking which is present from 36 weeks PMA onwards.

to the specifics of the situation. The ample spontaneous activity especially prepares the nervous system for the accurate and integrated use of afferent, perceptual information to adapt motor behaviour in a later phase. For instance, the spontaneous motor behaviour assists the fine-tuning of the genetically based structure of the somatosensory cortex (Hadders-Algra 2018c). In short, in the phase of primary variability, motor behaviour is characterized by variation with no or marginal adaptation (Hadders-Algra 2010, 2018c).

At a certain point in time, especially after the age of three months post-term, when the transient subplate has dissolved in the primary sensorimotor cortices, the phase of secondary or adaptive variability starts (Figure 2.3; Hadders-Algra 2018a, 2018c). In this phase, the nervous system clearly uses the afferent information produced by behaviour and experience for selection of the motor behaviour that fits the situation best (Edelman 1989, Hadders-Algra 2010, 2018c). In other words, the infant learns to adapt its motor behaviour, or – in terms of the IMP – adaptability emerges. The age at which the infant masters adaptability is function specific (Figure 2.3). For instance, in the development of reaching movements of the arm, it generally emerges between 5 and 13 months, and in the development of fine manipulation, it emerges at eight months and is accomplished by almost 90% of infants at 18 months (Heineman et al. 2010b, Chapter 8). These two examples illustrate that the development of adaptability is characterized – just as the development of motor milestones is (Touwen 1976) – by a large inter-individual variation. Despite all variation, infants generally have reached the first stages of secondary variability of all basic motor functions, such as sucking, reaching, grasping, postural control, and locomotion, in the second half of the second postnatal year. However, it takes until late adolescence before the secondary neural repertoire has achieved its adult configuration (Hadders-Algra 2010, 2018c).

The phase of secondary variability is characterized by movement selection, a process that is based on active trial-and-error experiences (experience-dependent development) (Greenough et al. 1987, Edelman 1993, Takahashi et al. 2013). This means that spontaneous (i.e., self-generated) motor behaviour with its associated sensorimotor experience plays a pivotal role (Hadders-Algra 2018c). Sensorimotor experience involves multimodal information: that is, the combined information from multiple sensory systems, such as the proprioceptive, haptic, visual, and auditory systems. The process of motor learning and selection from the repertoire is especially effective when the infant engages in play with others: for example, caregivers or siblings. The infant not only learns from his own trial-and-error attempts but also profits from the actions performed by others due to the neural mirroring mechanisms (Meltzoff et al. 2009, Hadders-Algra 2021a).

It is important to realize that motor development is not an isolated developmental phenomenon. Motor development is intertwined with sensory, cognitive, language, and social development (Bornstein et al. 2013, Adolph and Hoch 2019). For example, the infant's ability to move around via belly crawling allows him to explore the environment and to move to caregivers when being called, whereas reading a baby book with Mom not only invites the child to verbally communicate and improve his understanding of the world, but also encourages the child to produce pointing and page-turning movements.

NGST and atypical motor development

Atypical motor development may originate from genetic aberrations or adversities occurring during early development. Either aetiological pathway may result in a structural anomaly or lesion of the developing brain or in a different setting of specific neurotransmitter systems, such as the monoaminergic systems. In the following paragraphs, these two sequelae are addressed separately, but it should be kept in mind that lesions of the immature brain are often associated with changes in specific neurotransmitter systems (Kolb and Gibb 2007).

In terms of NGST, an early lesion of the brain, such as is present in children with CP, has two major consequences. First, the motor repertoire is reduced (Hadders-Algra 2010, Heineman et al. 2010a, 2011). In young infants, this means that the repertoire of movement combinations is reduced; in older infants and children, it implies the presence of a reduced repertoire of motor strategies. The repertoire reduction results in less varied and more stereotyped motor behaviour: that is, in reduced variation during both phases of variability. This aspect of motor behaviour is assessed in the IMP domain 'variation'. Second, during secondary variability, children with early lesions of the brain have impairments in the selection of the most appropriately adapted strategy out of the limited repertoire. This aspect of motor behaviour is assessed in the IMP domain 'adaptability'. The impaired capacity to adapt motor behaviour and to select the best solution has a threefold origin. First, the exploratory drive of children with early lesions of the brain is often reduced (Landry et al. 1993, Festante et al. 2019). This reduces the infant's opportunities for trial-and-error experience. Second, the limited ability to select the most efficient strategy from the repertoire is related to the deficits in the processing of sensory information that are virtually always present in children with early lesions of the brain. Third, the presence of a reduced repertoire may hamper strategy selection when the brain lesion has erased the typical best strategy, and the child is forced to select a 'second-best' strategy (Hadders-Algra 2010).

Our knowledge of alterations in neurotransmitter settings due to adversities in early human life is limited. Most is known about the effect of early physiological and/or psychological stress on the monoaminergic systems. Examples of early stress are low-risk preterm birth, intrauterine growth retardation, and maternal psychological stress during pregnancy. Animal data indicate that stress during early life gives rise to changes in serotonergic and noradrenergic activity in the cerebral cortex and alterations in dopaminergic activity in the striatum and prefrontal cortex (Braun et al. 2017). Animal research also demonstrates that the monoaminergic systems play a role in the adaptation of motor behaviour by coding sensory information to adjust activity in the motor cortex (Vitrac and Benoit-Marand 2017). Human studies indicate that stress during early life indeed is associated with a less optimal neurological condition in infancy and with less adaptive behaviour in later life (Kikkert et al. 2010, Braun et al. 2017). Together, these data suggest that stress during early life – via the pathway of an altered setting of the monoaminergic systems – may be associated with limited adaptability of motor behaviour (Hadders-Algra 2010).

Motor development

This section offers a concise overview of motor development in the first two years. Details on how the various motor skills evolve are provided in the chapters describing the IMP items (Chapters 4 to 9; see also Hadders-Algra 2018c).

The first movements arise early during foetal life: at seven weeks PMA, the foetus starts to produce small sideways movements of the head and/or trunk (Lüchinger et al. 2008). This means that the first movements emerge before the spinal reflex loops have been completed. This illustrates that intrinsic, patterned spontaneous activity is a quintessential property of neural tissue (Hadders-Algra 2018c). Soon thereafter, however, the afferent information associated with spontaneously generated movements assists the further sculpting of the brain. At eight weeks PMA, the limbs also start to participate in the movements. The movements are small, short in duration, and simple. One to two weeks later, at nine to ten weeks PMA, general movements with complexity and variation emerge. The foetus explores during the general movements all movement combinations of the various body joints (complexity) continuously over time (variation) (Hadders-Algra 2018b).

Soon after the emergence of the first movements, other movements are added to the foetal repertoire, such as isolated arm and leg movements, startles, stretches, periodic breathing movements, and sucking and swallowing movements. All movements continue to be present throughout pregnancy, with the general movements being the most frequently used movement pattern (de Vries and Fong 2006). The general movements persist until three to five months post-term, when they are gradually replaced by goal-directed activity.

In the following paragraphs, we outline the development of motor skills. However, it should be realized that this global summary does injustice to the large intra-individual and inter-individual variation of typical development and, thereby, to the variation underlying the IMP.

In the development of gross motor skills, two different components may be distinguished: (1) the ability to maintain a specific position, such as sitting and standing, and (2) the ability to move around: for instance, via rolling, crawling, and walking. Both types of activities depend strongly on postural control. The basic structural commands for postural control are present shortly after term age, but it takes many years for postural control to achieve its adult configuration. Postural control does not develop in a cranio-to-caudal direction as is often presumed; it develops from a varied use of postural muscles to a situation-specific selection of postural muscle activity (Hadders-Algra 2008, 2018c). The idea that the development of postural control follows a cranio-caudal order is presumably based on the observation that infants get increasingly better in coping with less postural support during sitting, standing, and walking. At early age, the young infant is only able to control a body part consisting of a few segments: the infant is able to balance the head while receiving full body support. With increasing age, the infant is able to master control of an increasing number of body segments; this allows the infant to sit, to stand, and to walk independently. A major transition in the organization of postural commands is the rapid increase in anticipatory postural control when the infant learns to walk independently. The development of both abilities is highly interrelated: a certain level of postural control allows the infant to explore walking abilities, whereas the probing walking behaviour feeds the postural control system with trial-and-error learning experiences (Boxum et al. 2019).

By and large, gross motor development is characterized by the following events (Hadders-Algra 2018c). Around three months, the infant is able to balance his head on his trunk, be it with some wobbling movements. From four to five months onwards, infants start to roll and to move around on their bellies (pivoting and belly crawling); this generally changes into crawling on all fours between 6 and 11 months of age. Meanwhile, infants learn to sit independently (mostly at six to nine months), to stand without support (mostly at 10 to 16 months), and – a bit later – to walk independently (mostly at 10 to 17 months).

Also, the development of manual skills is dependent on postural control and/or postural support. At around three months, infants start to play with their hands in the midline, and from four to five months onwards, they are able to reach towards and grasp an object. The infant's reaches consist of varied bilateral and unilateral movements with a unilateral preference. First one object can be held, but relatively soon thereafter, the infant can hold two objects (i.e., one in each hand). Between 6 and 12 months, unilateral reaches are increasingly preferred, with a varied use of the right and left side. From about 9 to 14 months, infants also learn to grasp an object while holding another object in the same hand. Over the first 18 months of life, the infant becomes increasingly able to fine-tune hand mobility to the form of the object. The use of the thumb and index finger especially becomes increasingly specialized. Early grasping behaviour consists mainly of full palmar grasps, but with increasing age, only the radial side of the hand is used (radial palmar grasp). At the end of the first year, the inferior pincer grasp (with extended thumb and flexed index finger) starts to dominate, after which the pincer grasp (with flexion of thumb and index finger) emerges (Hadders-Algra 2018c).

Concluding remarks

In brain and motor development, two phases can be distinguished: (1) the transient cortical subplate phase and (2) the permanent circuitries phase. The former is characterized by the presence of the cortical subplate in the primary sensory and motor cortices, implying that it ends at three months post-term, when the subplate in these areas has disappeared. In this phase, motor behaviour is characterized by variation with no or marginal adaptability. This is exemplified by the varied general movements. The phase in which the permanent circuitries dominate is the phase during which the brain is increasingly able to make sense of multimodal afferent information and the child develops specific motor skills. This phase is characterized by variation and an increasing ability to adapt motor behaviour to environmental constraints. In other words, motor behaviour is characterized by variation and increasing adaptability.

The knowledge that infants who have experienced adversities during early life may present with limited variation and limited adaptability in motor behaviour inspired us to develop the IMP, with its two novel domains, 'variation' and 'adaptability'.

Note

1 Note that, in the IMP manual, the word *variability* refers to the two developmental phases of the NGST, whereas the word *variation* is used to denote the infant's movement repertoire.

3 Design, performance, and psychometric properties of the IMP

Design of the IMP

The IMP is a video-based assessment of self-generated motor behaviour in infants aged 3 to 18 months or, in the assessment of infants experiencing a developmental delay, until the infant has achieved the ability to walk independently for a couple of months. The IMP provides information on the quality of the infant's movements especially, but it also furnishes information on the infant's level of motor performance. It is a discriminative, evaluative, and predictive measurement. The method has been developed for health care professionals working in the field of early detection of developmental disorders and early intervention, in particular for paediatric physiotherapists, paediatric occupational therapists, neonatologists, neuropaediatricians, and developmental paediatricians.

During the IMP assessment. motor behaviour is assessed in supine, prone, sitting, standing, and walking positions; in addition, reaching, grasping, and manipulation of objects are assessed. The examination takes place in a semi-structured play situation. This means that the examiner guides the infant through various play situations in different positions in order to give the child the opportunity to generate by himself the different types of motor behaviour. If the child does not show a certain motor behaviour spontaneously, the examiner tries to elicit it by presenting attractive toys to the infant. In the upcoming chapters, we provide specific guidelines on how to perform the IMP assessment in the various positions.

The IMP video assessment usually takes about 15 minutes, but more time may be required if the infant has behavioural issues, such as shyness or irritability. The scoring of the IMP video and the calculation of the IMP scores take, on average, another ten minutes.

The IMP consists of five motor domains: variation, adaptability, symmetry, fluency, and performance. The domains variation and adaptability are based on the NGST (see Chapter 2).

- *Variation* (25 items): this domain assesses the size of the motor repertoire. The motor repertoire consists of all combinations of movements possible in the various joints partaking in the movement. For instance, during reaching, the movements in the shoulders (flexion, extension, abduction, adduction, endorotation, exorotation), elbows (flexion, extension, supination, pronation), and wrists (flexion, extension, abduction, adduction) are taken into account. The variation items are scored dichotomously: insufficient variation or sufficient variation.

- *Adaptability* (15 items): this domain assesses the ability to select motor strategies out of the repertoire. The items are scored dichotomously: the majority of movements show signs of adaptive selection or the majority of movements are not adaptive.
- *Symmetry* (10 items): this domain assesses the presence of asymmetries in motor behaviour. The items are scored as strong, moderate, or no/mild asymmetry. Strong asymmetries are those that strike the eye, and moderate asymmetries those that are frequently but not consistently observed. Mild asymmetries can only be detected by careful observation. Note that mild asymmetries and no asymmetries are assigned a similar score. This implies that a mild asymmetry on a specific item is considered typical behaviour (Straathof et al. 2020).
- *Fluency* (7 items): this domain evaluates movement fluency and the presence of tremors. The items are scored dichotomously: the majority of movements are fluent or not. The latter implies, for instance, the presence of jerky, abrupt, stiff, or tremulous movements.
- *Performance* (23 items): in contrast to the other domains, this domain does not assess the quality of movements, but rather, the infant's motor achievements (milestones). The items of this domain are not scored in a standard way (i.e., similarly for all items), but scoring is adapted to the specific motor function, with multi-point scores ranging from 2 to 7.

In the domains of variation, adaptability, and fluency, the assessor needs to assign the overall impression of the infant's behaviour. It may happen that the assessor is in doubt which category to assign as the infant shows movements that are just (or just not) sufficiently varied, adaptive, or fluent. We recommend making the best fitting choice and letting the IMP design do the rest of the work: the final score of the domains does not depend on a single item but on a number of domain items. This implies that the system has a self-weighing character: that is, not meeting the criteria for one or two items does not have clinical significance. Only a significant reduction in domain score is clinically relevant (see Chapter 10).

The IMP generates five domain scores and a total score. These scores are computed with the help of the IMP app, which is available on the IMP's website at infantmotorprofile.com. In children over the age of six months, the total IMP score is calculated as the mean of the five domain scores. In children of six months and younger, the adaptability domain score is not taken into account in the total score as the ability to select strategies from the motor repertoire has a slow start and first begins to bloom after the age of six months (Heineman et al. 2010a). Details of the IMP calculation are provided in Box 3.1. The IMP items, including their scoring procedures, are described in Chapters 4 through 9.

Box 3.1   Calculation of the IMP scores – background details

On the basis of the 80 items, the five domain scores and the total IMP score are calculated. For the domain scores, only the items that have been assessed are taken into account. The items that are not assessed are assigned score 0 (see score form and Chapters 4 through 8); the 0 score signals to the IMP app calculator that the item is not taken into account in the computation of the scores.

The variation, adaptability, fluency, and symmetry domain scores are calculated as follows:

$$\text{Domain score (\%)} = \frac{\text{sum of item scores}}{(\text{number of assessed items}) \times \text{maximum score of items}}$$

The maximum score of the items is different for the various domains: for the items in the variation, adaptability, and fluency domains, the maximum score is 2; for the items in the symmetry domain, the maximum is 3.

In the calculation of the performance domain scores, the scores are weighted per item. That means, for instance, that if an item has 7 options (for example, item 14) and the infant received score 3, this contributes $3/7 = 0.43$ to the performance domain score. The weighted scores of all performance items are combined and divided by the number of assessed performance items, resulting in the performance domain score.

For infants older than six months, the adaptability domain score is calculated. This domain score is not calculated for younger infants as adaptability is only present to a limited extent in early infancy. As a result, the total IMP score is calculated as the mean of all five domain scores in infants older than six months and as the mean of four domains in infants six months old or younger as, in the latter group, no adaptability score is available.

Importantly, users of the IMP do not need to do these maths; the IMP app automatically calculates the IMP scores.

Implementation in clinical practice

Typical course of the IMP assessment

For young infants, the IMP assessment starts in a supine position on a thin mattress on the floor. In this position, the first three to five minutes of spontaneous movements are recorded, during which the child does not interact with the examiner or caregivers. Next, the examiner presents toys to the infant – who still lies supine – in order to assess head movements, reaching, grasping and manipulation, and rolling movements. In older children, the supine position is skipped as they usually promptly move out of this position (see Chapter 4).

The next part of the IMP assessment consists of the evaluation in the prone position. Motor behaviour of the head, arms, and legs is assessed, and crawling behaviour is examined. Next, motor behaviour in the sitting position is assessed; sitting may be supported or independent. In older infants, standing up, standing, and walking are assessed. In the older children, the IMP assessment is less structured as the children typically change position quite often during play.

In the last part of the IMP assessment, the child sits on the lap of the caregiver. The infant's reaching, grasping, and manipulation of objects are assessed by presenting toys. If, at the start of the IMP assessment, the child is very shy or reluctant to engage, it may be better to start the assessment with this part of the examination: that is, the assessment on the caregiver's lap. In this way, the child can get used to the testing situation while having secure support. Table 3.1 summarizes the recommendations on the practical procedures of the IMP.

Table 3.1 Recommendations on the practical procedures of the IMP

Position of the infant and actions of the examiner

Supine: in young infants or infants who are not able to move around in the room
- Start with three to five minutes of spontaneous motility without interaction, child in the supine position on thin mattress on the floor.
- Elicit head movements in different directions by presenting toys.
- Elicit reaching, grasping, and manipulation behaviour of arms and hands by presenting toys. Important: present toys in various positions and directions; present toys of different sizes and shapes. Use especially toys that easily fit in one hand of the infant. First one toy is presented, then a second toy, and, if possible, a third toy. Do not put toys in the infant's hand. Do not touch the hands of the infant.
- Elicit rolling behaviour from the supine to the prone position by presenting a toy just out of the infant's reach in the arm area between 90 and 180 degrees of shoulder abduction. Assess both sides.

Prone: all infants
- Minimum one minute in total; if difficult, assess small stints of 20 to 30 seconds.
- Place young infant in the prone position with shoulders in adduction and both elbows in flexion with the hands approximately in line with the ears.
- Older infants spontaneously adopt prone position.
- Assess capacity to lift head and look around by presenting toys or the examiner's face.
- Elicit arm and hand movements in the prone position by presenting toys in various directions and at various distances on and above the support surface in front of the infant.
- Elicit progression in the prone position with the help of toys (ball, car, train): pivoting or (abdominal) crawling. In older infants: elicit crawling by the crawling of the examiner or caregiver, or build a tunnel with a small table or chairs and move interesting objects through it. In infants who show (abdominal) crawling, at least two instances of a few crawling 'steps' are needed to obtain IMP scores.

Sitting: on the floor or on a mattress, all ages
- Young infants are placed in sitting position (e.g., by the pull-to-sit manoeuvre).
- Assess head control and head movements in supported sitting position by presenting a toy or the face of the examiner.
- Assess sitting behaviour by giving as little support as possible, gradually lowering the supporting hands and seeing whether the infant can sit independently.
- If the infant sits independently, assess weight shifts and trunk rotations by presenting toys in various positions; assess rotation to both sides.
- In older children: assess the ability to sit up and down independently and change positions (e.g., prone to sitting, standing to sitting). Take care to have multiple trials of getting into the sitting position.
- If the child shows only W sitting (between knees with legs in W form): also sit the infant on his buttocks and evaluate the infant's ability to shift weight and to rotate.
- In older infants: assess reaching and grasping of toys in the sitting position on the floor as described in the section that follows on reaching, grasping, and manipulation. Note that this does not mean that assessment on the lap may be omitted.

Standing and walking: only ≥ age six months
- Assess for several minutes, depending on age and functional capacities of child.
- Elicit standing-up behaviour by putting toys on small chair or table; elicit sitting-down behaviour by putting the toys on the floor. Repeat this a few times.
- If a child who is at least six months old is not able to stand up by himself, assess the ability to stand with help: put the infant in standing position and see whether he puts his weight on his legs (or let the caregiver do this).
- If the infant is able to stand independently the ability to rotate the trunk is tested by presentation of toys in various directions on both sides of the body and at various heights.
- If the infant is able to stand and walk independently, elicit various ways of standing up and sitting down.

- If the child is not able to walk independently, assess walking while holding the hands of the caregiver or assessor: first two hands, then see if the infant can walk with the support of one hand. Cruising alongside a small table or chair may serve as an alternative to walking with the support of two hands.
- If the child is able to walk independently, assess behaviour walking across the room. Elicit this by presenting toys, and encourage the child to bring the toys to the caregiver. Challenge the child to walk on the mattress and to avoid objects on the floor.

Reaching, grasping, and manipulation of objects: on the lap of the caregiver, all ages
- Sit the infant on the lap of a caregiver seated on a chair or sofa, but not on the floor. Inform the caregiver that the infant needs to sit comfortably, but give no specific instructions on postural support.
- Elicit reaching or prereaching behaviour by presenting a toy, first in the midline at arm-length distance. If the infant grasps and manipulates the toy for some time, retrieve the toy and repeat this in various positions in space.
- If the infant is able to grasp one toy, present a second and third and test how many objects the infant can hold at a time. Present the toys sequentially, not simultaneously.
- Vary with different toy sizes and shapes to elicit different hand and finger movements. Use especially toys that easily fit in one hand of the infant. Include a small object to elicit pincer grasp on both sides.
- With very shy infants, you can start the assessment of reaching and grasping on the caregiver's lap, so the child can adapt slowly to the examiner and the circumstances.

Behavioural state and movement quantity

During the entire assessment, the infant's behavioural state is monitored as the behavioural state has a significant impact on the results of a neurodevelopmental examination (Prechtl 1977). For instance, crying induces a reduction in movement variation and promotes stereotypes (Hadders-Algra 2004). However, in general, it is easy to have the infant in an active, alert, and cooperative behavioural state as infants like the IMP play.

To monitor the effect of the behavioural state and that of other conditions that may affect the infant's behaviour, these factors (behavioural state, health condition, and others) are recorded at the end of the IMP score form (or at the end of the IMP app). These additional observations, including the observation of the quantity of the infant's movements, are not part of the IMP score.

The quantity of movements is recorded as typical (++), hypokinetic (+) (i.e., moving so little that the assessor gets uneasy as so little happens per unit of time), or hyperkinetic (+++) (i.e., moving so much that it is challenging to manage the play with the child).

The majority of infants have a typical movement quantity. The quantity of movements provides information on the amount of the infant's self-generated movement experience. It may also help explain the infant's scores in the domains of adaptability and performance.

Requirements

The IMP assessment can be performed in different settings and situations, such as a consulting room, a physiotherapy practice, or the child's home. In the latter case, it is important to create sufficient space in the room for the child to move around freely.

The IMP assessment is recorded on video and, scoring is performed at a later time on the basis of the video. Any video camera will do, but we recommend a digital video camera placed on a tripod as this results in good-quality images. Ideally, two assessors are involved, so one person can handle the video camera while the other person is engaged in the IMP play with the infant. However, a single person is certainly able to perform an IMP assessment. The assessor first takes care that the camera on the tripod is positioned in such a way that it covers the space where the examination is performed; then she performs the assessment.

Besides the camera and tripod, the IMP assessment requires a thin mattress on which the infant may lie or sit (or over which the infant may stumble or adaptively step) and a set of toys. Recommended toys are generally commercially available: for instance, small puppets, rings, rattles, balls, and toy cars (Figure 3.1). For the assessment of reaching, grasping, and manipulation, care is taken to use objects that are about the size of the infant's hand. Note that many commercially available infant rings and rattles are considerably larger and thus not adequate for the evaluation of reaching, grasping, and manipulation. For the evaluation of the inferior pincer grasp and pincer grasp, it is recommended to have objects that require this behaviour for proper manipulation. Examples are a chest of drawers with small knobs, puzzles with small knobs, or a retractable measurement tape with a case (Figure 3.1). To elicit standing-up behaviour, a big box, small chair, sofa, or table can be used.

The IMP is recorded on the IMP assessment form (Figure 3.2) available from the URL www.routledge.com/cw/hadders-algra or in the IMP app. The app automatically generates the IMP domain scores and the total IMP score. The app can be found on the website of the IMP manual at infantmotorprofile.com.

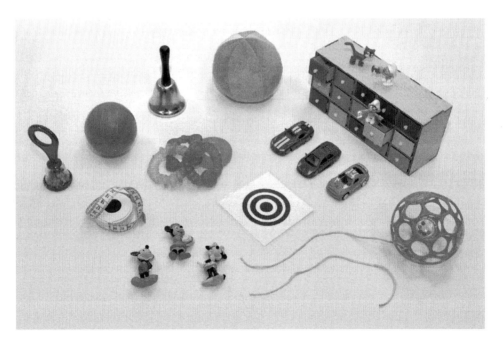

Figure 3.1 Recommended material for the IMP assessment. It includes rings in the size of the infant's hand, small puppets, cars, balls, a bell, and objects that elicit the pincer grasp, such as the knobs of the chest of drawers, the tail of the cat, or the retractable measurement tape.

Infant Motor Profile

Developmental Neurology
University Medical Center Groningen, The Netherlands

Participant ID number:

Assessor:

(Corrected) Age: ♂ / ♀

Assessment date:

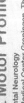

Supine

Assessment of supine items

A ☐ assessed, go to item 1
NA ☐ not assessed, go to item 22

1. Control of head movements [P]

1 ☐ cannot control head movements
2 ☐ can control head movements to a limited extent
3 ☐ can control head movements

2. Variation in head movements [V]

1 ☐ insufficient variation
2 ☐ sufficient variation

3. Adaptability of head movements [A]

majority of movements:
1 ☐ no adaptive selection
2 ☐ adaptive selection

4. Position of head, prevailing head position to one side [S]

1 ☐ strongly prevailing head position to the ☐ R / ☐ L
2 ☐ moderately prevailing head position to the ☐ R / ☐ L
3 ☐ no or mildly prevailing head position to one side

5. Posture, presence of ATNR [V]

1 ☐ frequently occurring or obligatory ATNR
2 ☐ no ATNR or occasionally non-obligatory ATNR

6. Posture, presence of hyperextension of neck and trunk [V]

1 ☐ frequently occurring or persistent hyperextension
2 ☐ no or rarely hyperextension

7. Manipulative behaviour of hands and fingers [P]

1 ☐ no manipulative behaviour
2 ☐ manipulates clothes, with hands in midline, on knees or feet; plays with hands at mouth

8. Variation in arm movements [V]

1 ☐ insufficient variation
2 ☐ sufficient variation

9. Variation in finger movements [V]

1 ☐ insufficient variation
2 ☐ sufficient variation

10. Tilting of pelvis [P]

1 ☐ no tilting of pelvis
2 ☐ tilts pelvis, but not in such a way that hands may be able to touch knees
3 ☐ tilts pelvis in such a way that hands may be able to touch knees
4 ☐ hands play with feet

11. Variation in leg movements [V]

1 ☐ insufficient variation
2 ☐ sufficient variation

12. Variation in toe movements [V]

1 ☐ insufficient variation
2 ☐ sufficient variation

13. Rolling from the supine into the prone position [P]

1 ☐ no turning or rolling attempts
2 ☐ makes 'wiggling' movements with the pelvis, but does not roll to side
3 ☐ rolls to side, unilaterally ☐ R / ☐ L
4 ☐ rolls to side, bilaterally
5 ☐ turns unilaterally into prone ☐ R / ☐ L
6 ☐ turns bilaterally into prone

14. Reaching, grasping, and manipulation of objects [P]

1 ☐ does not reach, does not show prereaching movements
2 ☐ does not reach, but shows prereaching movements
3 ☐ reaches towards object but does not grasp it
4 ☐ reaches towards, grasps and holds object, but does not manipulate object
5 ☐ reaches towards, holds and manipulates 1 object
6 ☐ reaches towards, holds and manipulates 2 objects
7 ☐ reaches towards and holds ≥ 3 objects

15. Reaching, grasping, and manipulating objects: presence of asymmetry [S]

0 ☐ no prereaching or reaching movements (item 14, score 1)
1 ☐ strong asymmetry, ☐ R / ☐ L worst side
2 ☐ moderate asymmetry, ☐ R / ☐ L worst side
3 ☐ no or mild asymmetry

Figure 3.2 First page of the IMP–score form

Psychometric properties of the IMP

An important part in the process of the development of a new instrument is the assessment of its psychometric properties, especially reliability, validity, and responsiveness to change (Sargent 2021). Reliability is the reproducibility of scores when the same assessment is scored by different assessors (inter-rater reliability) or at different moments in time by the same assessor (intra-rater reliability). Also, various forms of validity can be distinguished. Construct validity of an instrument is the extent to which the instrument measures what it is intended to measure – the construct of interest – in this case, neuromotor condition. Concurrent validity refers to the instrument's capacity to generate scores that are comparable – but not identical – to those of other instruments assessing comparable constructs. Predictive validity describes the instrument's capacity to predict later developmental outcomes.

The psychometric properties of the IMP have been studied in various clinical populations and in the so-called IMP-SINDA project. The IMP-SINDA project was designed to collect norm data of the IMP and the Standardized Infant NeuroDevelopmental Assessment (SINDA) (Hadders-Algra et al. 2019, 2020) in a group of infants representative of the Dutch population. The data were collected between January 2017 and March 2019 in a sample of 1,700 infants aged two to 18 months born in the three Northern provinces of the Netherlands. The sample consisted of 100 infants of each age (100 two-month-olds, 100 three-month-olds, etc.). Participants were recruited via well-baby clinics, nurseries, and mailings. Each infant was assessed once. Exclusion criteria were severe congenital abnormalities, such as severe congenital heart disease with low oxygen level, which precluded assessment, and caregivers having insufficient understanding of the Dutch language to give informed consent. The assessments took place in the University Medical Center Groningen or at the child's home. The infants were representative of the Dutch population in terms of maternal education, ethnicity, sex, and preterm birth (see Table 3.2) (Straathof et al. 2020, Wu et al. 2020a). The data of the IMP-SINDA project were also used to create percentile curves (see Chapter 10).

Table 3.2 Background characteristics of children participating in the IMP norm study (n=1,700)

Background characteristic	
Sex: male/female, n (%)	888 (52%)/812 (48%)
Gestational age (weeks; SD; range)	39.4 (1.8; 27.3–42.4)
Preterm birth <37 weeks, n (%)	138 (8%)
Twins, n (%)	60 (3.5%)
Birth weight (grams; SD; range)	3,440 (580; 1,120–5,020)
Birth weight <p10, n (%)	191 (11%)
Educational level mother high[a], n (%)	790 (47%)
Educational level father high[a,b], n (%)	693 (41%)
Ethnicity mother: Dutch/non-Dutch, n (%)	1,548 (91%)/152 (9%)
Ethnicity father: Dutch/non-Dutch	1,516 (89%)/184 (11%)[c]

a University education or vocational college
b Missing data for n=50, of whom n=28 father donor, no data available
c Missing data for n=28, father donor, no data available

Note that for the calculation of the IMP norm curves, the data of the two-month-old infants were also used.

Reliability

Four studies assessed the reliability of the IMP. Three of them addressed intra-rater reliability. Intra-rater reliability of the total IMP score and the performance domain score was high (Spearman's rho or intraclass correlation coefficients [ICC] >0.85). It was satisfactory for the other domain scores (median values across studies: variation rho 0.80, ICC 0.82; adaptability rho 0.80, ICC 0.78; symmetry rho 0.60, ICC 0.61, fluency rho 0.60, ICC 0.84) (Heineman et al. 2008, Hecker et al. 2016, Tveten et al. 2020). Inter-rater reliability was assessed in all four reliability studies. Again, reliability of the total IMP score and the performance domain was high (Spearman's rho and ICC >0.85) and satisfactory for the other domain scores (median values across studies: variation rho 0.70, ICC 0.72, adaptability rho 0.80, ICC 0.66, symmetry rho 0.40, ICC 0.40, fluency rho 0.70, ICC 0.66) (Heineman et al. 2008, Heineman et al. 2013, Hecker et al. 2016, Tveten et al. 2020).

Validity

The construct validity of the IMP was evaluated in a mixed sample of high and low risk infants and in the 1,600 infants of the IMP-SINDA project aged 3 to 18 months. A proper construct of the IMP implies that IMP scores decrease in infants with a history of perinatal adversities, such as preterm birth and neonatal complications, including a lesion of the brain. In addition, it implies that the total IMP score and the adaptability and performance domain scores increase with increasing age. The study in the mixed sample indicates that the total IMP score decreases with decreasing gestational age at birth, the presence of a significant brain lesion, and lower social class and increases with increasing age at assessment (Heineman et al. 2010a, 2010b). In the infants representative of the Dutch population, low total IMP scores were predominantly associated with maternal smoking during pregnancy and a non-optimal start after birth. Table 3.3 summarizes the associations between perinatal and social factors on the one hand and low IMP domain scores (<5th percentile) on the other hand. The data confirm the construct validity of the IMP.

The concurrent validity of the IMP was demonstrated in a mixed sample of high- and low-risk infants assessed at 4, 6, 10, 12, and 18 months. The total IMP scores correlated fairly to moderately with the Alberta Infant Motor Scale (AIMS) scores (r=0.37–0.54), with the performance domain of the IMP having the strongest correlations with the AIMS scores (Heineman et al. 2013). At all ages tested, total IMP scores were also associated with the infant's neurological condition assessed with the Touwen infant neurological examination, with infants with a normal neurological condition having higher IMP scores than those with abnormal neurological conditions (Heineman et al. 2013). Also, four of the five IMP domain scores (variation, symmetry, fluency, and performance) were at all ages associated with neurological condition. The adaptability domain was associated with neurological condition at 10 and 12 months and only marginally at 18 months (Heineman et al. 2013).

In the infants representative of the Dutch population, low total IMP scores and all domain scores were strongly associated with atypical scores on the neurological scale of the SINDA (Table 3.4), confirming the concurrent validity of the IMP and SINDA.

Predictive validity was assessed in three studies. The first study addressed the ability of the IMP to predict CP in a mixed sample of high- and low-risk infants. The infants had been longitudinally assessed with the IMP throughout infancy. The study indicated a high predictive ability of total IMP scores for CP (area under receiver operating characteristic curve [ROC] 0.89–0.99, depending on age, CI's ranging from 0.75–1.00 to 0.97–1.00).

Table 3.3 Associations between perinatal and socio-economic factors and low IMP scores in the IMP-SINDA norm population, logistic regression analyses, n=1,600 infants

IMP score < 5th percentile	Variable	OR	95% CI
IMP domain scores			
Variation	maternal hypertension	2.055	1.094–3.858
Adaptability[a,b]	–	–	–
Symmetry < 6 mo	–	–	–
Symmetry ≥ 6 mo	maternal hypertension	2.347	1.139–4.839
	ethnicity mother	2.366	1.073–5.214
Fluency	maternal gestational diabetes	3.427	1.374–8.547
Performance	high educational level of the father[c]	0.559	0.315–0.991
Total IMP score			
Total IMP score	smoking during pregnancy	2.351	1.144–4.831
	non-optimal start	2.439	1.187–5.014

OR = odds ratio

a   Infants >6 mo, n=1,200
b   Below P15 as no 5th percentile could be calculated for the adaptability domain
c   University or vocational college

Table 3.4 Concurrent validity of IMP and SINDA: associations between low IMP scores (<5th percentile) and atypical SINDA neurological score in the IMP-SINDA norm population (odds ratio and confidence interval)

IMP score	n		SINDA neurological score		OR (95% CI)
			atypical[a]	typical	
IMP domain scores					
Variation	1,000	<P5	14	49	5.940 (3.045–11.587)
		≥P5	43	894	
Adaptability	600	<P5	5	27	3.262 (1.207–8.817)
		≥P5	52	916	
Symmetry <6 mo	300	<P5	4	4	10.231 (2.416–43.321)
		≥P5	26	266	
Symmetry ≥6 mo	700	<P5	5	43	3.330 (1.202–9.225)
		≥P5	22	630	
Fluency	1,000	<P5	7	24	5.361 (2.204–13.038)
		≥P5	50	919	
Performance	1,000	<P5	8	36	4.113 (1.815–9.323)
		≥P5	49	907	
Total IMP score					
Total IMP score	1,000	<P5	11	33	6.594 (3.134–13.875)
		≥P5	46	910	

n = number of infants; note that SINDA scores are only available for the infants aged 3–12 months, as SINDA's upper age limit is 12 months

a   Atypical SINDA neurological score means a score of ≤21 points (out of a total of 28 points). It is associated with a highly increased risk of developmental disorders (Hadders-Algra et al. 2019, 2020).

The variation and performance domains contributed most to IMP's predictive ability (Heineman et al. 2011). However, it is important to note there was some overlap in the IMP scores of infants who later were and were not diagnosed with CP, indicating that prediction was not perfect (see also Chapter 10).

The other two studies on IMP's predictive validity were performed in a relatively low-risk sample of 195 children born to parents with reduced fertility, who were or were not treated with in vitro fertilization. It was found that IMP scores throughout infancy were related to cognitive, neurological, and behavioural function at school age: higher adaptability scores were associated with higher IQ and more optimal neurological function, higher performance scores with higher IQ, and lower variation and fluency scores with more internalizing behavioural problems (Heineman et al. 2018, Wu et al. 2020b).

Responsiveness to change

Responsiveness to change is the ability of an instrument to detect clinically important changes over time. Within the field of neuromotor development, an instrument's responsiveness to change especially implies the ability of the instrument to detect the effect of early intervention. Four studies indicated that the IMP is, indeed, a responsive instrument. The first was the study of Hielkema et al. (2011), which evaluated in infants at very high risk of CP the effect of the early intervention program Coping with and Caring for Infants with Special Needs (COPCA), a family-centred programme (Dirks et al. 2011). It demonstrated that the application of specific COPCA components was associated with better IMP scores (especially better total scores and adaptability scores). The other three studies were performed in groups of very preterm infants at low-to-moderate risk of developmental disorders. One study also evaluated the effect of COPCA. It demonstrated that the infants who had received COPCA had significantly higher IMP scores than the infants in the control group, who had received typical infant physiotherapy. The effect was found in particular in the IMP variation and performance domains (Akhbari Ziegler et al. 2020). The other two studies evaluated the effect of the CareToy system. Both studies indicated that the IMP was able to detect significant differences between the experimental CareToy group and the standard-care group, with the study infants having higher total scores and variation and performance scores (Sgandurra et al. 2016, 2017).

Introduction to the chapters with the description of the items

The following six chapters contain the descriptions of the IMP items: Chapter 4 describes the assessment while supine, Chapter 5 the assessment while prone, Chapter 6 the assessment while sitting, Chapter 7 the assessment while standing and walking, Chapter 8 the assessment of reaching, grasping, and manipulation while sitting on the caregiver's lap, and Chapter 9 addresses items that are assessed during the entire IMP assessment. The items are illustrated with figures and videos. The videos are available from the URL www.routledge.com/cw/hadders-algra. For the items that are age dependent, the age dependency is illustrated with the data of the infants representative of the Dutch population (IMP-SINDA project). This holds true especially for the items in the adaptability and performance domains.

4 Assessment of motor behaviour while supine

Procedure

For young infants, the assessment usually starts in the supine position (Figure 4.1). The infant is placed in the supine position on a thin mattress on the floor. The mattress should not have a toy-like structure: that is, have graspable structures as part of its construction. The supine assessment starts with an observation of the infant's spontaneous motor behaviour. This observation lasts for three to five, minutes during which the infant does not interact with the assessor or caregiver. This implies that the examiner and caregiver avoid attracting the infant's attention. Preferably, the caregiver sits or stands at some distance from the infant in a neutral position with respect to the infant's head in order to prevent a side preference of the head. If the infant sucks on a hand for more than a minute, we suggest bringing the infant's hand into another position. You may repeat this procedure once, but if the infant continues to suck on the hand, accept the sucking behaviour (and the resulting non-optimal testing condition).

During the first three to five minutes, no toys are used. Care is also taken that no toys are within reach of the infant. During this time, the infant's self-initiated activities, which are assessed in items 5 through 12, are evaluated. This also implies that the scores of items 5 through 12 are based on these first three to five minutes and that the infant's performance on these items during toy presentation in the supine position is *not* taken into account. Generally, a period of three minutes provides sufficient information to score items 5 through 12. Some infants, however, take their time before really starting to move; for these infants, the initial assessment time is extended to five minutes.

After the first three to five minutes, during which the infant's self-initiated movements in the absence of toys and the absence of interaction with the assessor is assessed, toys are used to evaluate goal-directed movements in the supine position. The goal-directed movements consist of movements of the head; the infant's ability to reach, grasp, and manipulate objects in the supine position; and the infant's ability to roll into the prone position (items 1–4 and 13–20).

In general, young infants who have been put into the supine position will remain in this position. This means that it is easy to record five minutes of spontaneous, self-initiated movements of young infants in the supine position. However, older infants do not stay in the supine position for prolonged periods as they prefer to play in a prone position, sitting, or standing and walking. The minimum duration of spontaneous, self-initiated movements in the supine position needed to assess the supine items 5 to 12 is about three minutes. If an infant turns to the prone position before having been in the supine position for three minutes, the infant is put once again into the supine position at

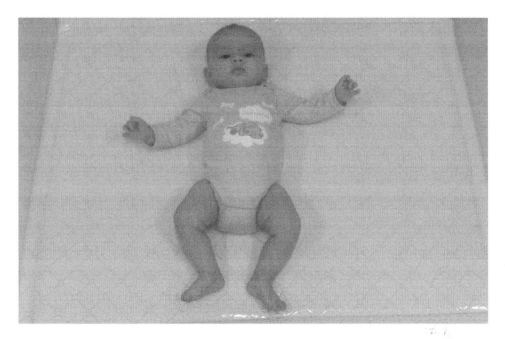

Figure 4.1 Assessment in supine: starting situation

a moment that suits the infant and the assessor. In this way, the minimum of three minutes of self-initiated movements in the supine position may be recorded.

Older infants generally do not stay very long in the supine position. As a result, motor behaviour in the supine position cannot be assessed. In this case, the 'not assessed' box is ticked, telling the calculator of the IMP app to assign the maximum score to the performance items 1, 7, 10, and 13 for the calculation of the domain and total scores. For children who walk independently, the supine section is skipped (tick the 'not assessed' box). Some children who are able to roll and crawl do remain in the supine position when put there. They may look around but refrain from further activity, as if they are waiting for things to happen. In these cases, the supine position also should be recorded as 'not assessed'.

During the period of the first three to five minutes of spontaneous, self-initiated movements, the assessor pays specific attention to the movements of the infant's head. If, after this time, it is still unclear to what extent the infant is able to control his head movements, the assessor tries to elicit specific, self-generated head movements in various directions. The movements may be elicited by the presentation of an attractive toy or by means of movements of the examiner's face from a distance of about 30 centimeters from the infant's face. Young infants have a strong preference for looking at the human faces (Johnson et al. 2015). In case of doubts about the infant's visual abilities, auditory cues (the examiner's voice, a bell, or a rattle) may be used to elicit head movements.

When sufficient information has been collected on the infant's ability to move his head (during the three to five minutes of spontaneous, self-initiated movements or during the specific assessment of the movement abilities of the head), reaching, grasping, and

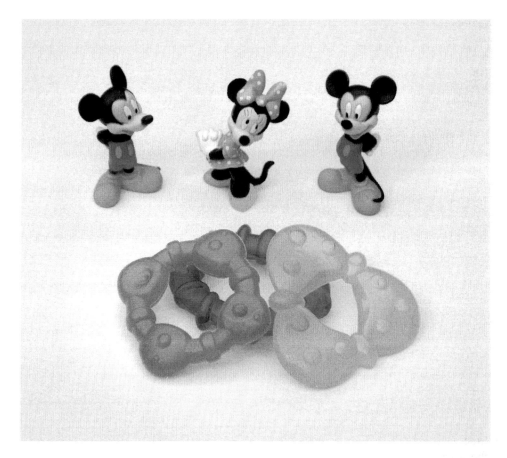

Figure 4.2 Objects used to assess reaching, grasping, and manipulation while supine

manipulation in the supine position is assessed. To this end, the assessor presents relatively small, attractive toys to the infant (relatively small means about the size of the infant's hand) (see Figure 4.2).

The presentation of the objects starts in an easy position (i.e., in the midline within reaching distance with an object that is easy to grasp – e.g., a simple ring with a diameter of about 6 cm) (see Figure 4.3). Reaching distance implies that the toy is not presented too close to the infant's face. The infant is verbally encouraged to grasp the object. The assessor patiently keeps the object still in space and waits for the infant's actions. The assessor does not move the object while waiting for the infant to reach; otherwise, it is difficult for the infant to determine target position. Therefore, no dangling objects are presented. When the infant has grasped an object, some time is allowed for object manipulation. Next, a second toy is presented. Again, the infant is given ample time to find his own solution for getting it. If the infant is able to handle two objects, the infant is offered two objects several times in succession. Thereafter, the assessor evaluates whether the infant is able to grasp an additional third object while holding two other ones. For the

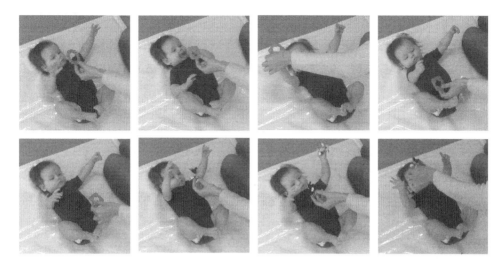

Figure 4.3 Assessment of reaching, grasping, and manipulation while supine. The assessment starts with the presentation of a simple object in the midline at reaching distance. To evaluate how many objects the infant can handle, objects are presented sequentially in the easy midline position. To assess variation and adaptability of arm and hand movements, the objects are placed at various positions in space and object form is varied.

evaluation of reaching, grasping, and manipulation, it is important that the infant's face and eyes (visual attention) are clearly recorded on video as well.

When the assessor has determined how many objects the infant can handle at a time (performance item 14), the focus of the assessment shifts to the evaluation of the variation and adaptability of the infant's arms and hands. To this end, the toys are presented one by one at a distance of about the length of the infant's arm (and not beyond!) and at various positions in space. Several times, the object is also placed closer to the infant's body. The spatial variation is needed in order to assess the infant's repertoire of arm and hand movements (variation) and ability to adapt reaching movements to the specifics of the condition (adaptability). To assess variation and adaptability of hand and finger movements, a variety of toys are used. First, simple rings are presented, followed by the presentation of more complex objects, such as small puppets (Figure 4.3).

When sufficient information on reaching, grasping, and manipulation has been collected, the infant's ability to roll into the prone position is assessed. To this end, attractive toys are presented just out of the infant's reach in the arm area between 90 and 180 degrees of shoulder abduction. First one direction is tested, then the other. If the infant rolls into the prone position, the infant is returned to the supine position in order to evaluate rolling abilities to the other side.

To wrap up, the scoring of the items 5 through 12 is entirely based on at least three minutes of spontaneous, self-initiated movements of the infant in the supine position without interference by the assessor. Items 1 through 4 and 13 through 20 generally require assessor activity for proper evaluation. For an example of the assessment in supine position, see Video 4.1.

1. Control of head movements (P)

Control of head movements while supine refers to the ability of the infant to master the movements of the head in this position. This item is assessed on the basis of behaviour during the first three to five minutes of spontaneous, self-initiated movements and – if these first minutes do not supply sufficient information – on the basis of the infant's behaviour in response to the presentation of an interesting object or the face of the assessor (Videos 4.2, 4.3, and 4.4).

1 = cannot control head movements
2 = can control head movements to a limited extent
3 = can control head movements

Score 1   The infant does not turn his head to the midline or in other directions. This means that the infant also maintains his head in one position when challenged to turn it in another direction.

Score 2   The infant has some capacity to turn his head and to maintain it in a limited number of positions, but he does not turn his head in all directions and does not maintain it in any desired position (Video 4.3).

Score 3   The infant turns his head in any desired direction and maintains it in any desired position. A score 3 does not necessarily imply that the infant is able to put his ear on the support surface on both sides (Video 4.2).

Note: the 'control of head movements' is based on the overall performance (while supine); this means that in this performance item, the general principle of the performance (P) domain, 'score the best performance observed', is not applied.

Figure 4.4 shows the development of the control of head movements in the norm population. At the youngest IMP age of three months, none of the infants entirely lacks

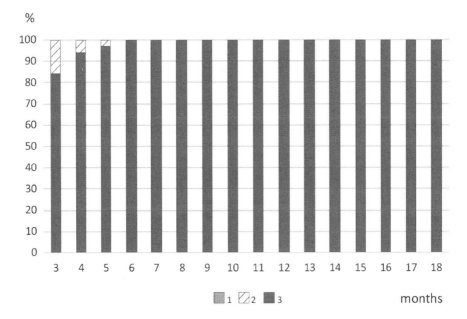

Figure 4.4 Development of the control of head movements while supine in the norm population (item 1). Each bar represents 100 infants; infants who could not be assessed anymore in supine automatically got assigned score 3. The numbers in the legends denote the scores of the item.

control of his head movements, and more than 80% already achieve score 3: 'can control head movements'. At six months of age, all infants have a fully developed control of their head movements while supine.

2.   Variation in head movements (V)

The size of the repertoire of head movements is assessed. This item is assessed on the basis of behaviour during the first three to five minutes of spontaneous, self-initiated movements and – if these first minutes do not supply sufficient information – on the basis of the infant's behaviour in response to presentation of an interesting object or the face of the assessor.

> 1 = insufficient variation
> 2 = sufficient variation

Score 1   The infant shows a limited repertoire of head movements, implying that the head is moved in a limited number of directions (Video 4.3).
Score 2   The infant shows movements of the head in various directions (e.g., to the right, to the left, retroflexion, and lateroflexion movements). In general, infants do not largely anteflex or retroflex their head in the supine position (Video 4.3).

3.   Adaptability of head movements (A)

Adaptability of head movements refers to the infant's ability to select in each situation the most appropriate head movement. This item is assessed on the basis of behaviour during the first three to five minutes of spontaneous, self-initiated movements and – if these first minutes do not supply sufficient information – on the basis of the infant's behaviour in response to presentation of an interesting object or the face of the assessor.

> 1 = majority of movements: no adaptive selection
> 2 = majority of movements: adaptive selection

Score 1   The infant does not or only occasionally selects the most appropriate motor strategy out of his repertoire of head movements for specific situations. The infant may explore various head movements, but he does not consistently move his head efficiently in a desired direction. Score 1 is also assigned if the infant has a seriously reduced movement repertoire consisting of only one strategy (Video 4.3).
Score 2   In general, the infant is able to choose the most appropriate and efficient motor strategy out of his motor repertoire for specific situations most of the time. For instance, the infant is able to turn his head efficiently at the right moment to the right spot: for example, to an attractive object (Video 4.3). Note that it is also possible to show adaptive motor behaviour when the movement repertoire (variation) is reduced. For instance, if an infant has a reduced motor repertoire consisting of a limitation in turning his head to the left side, a score 2 is given if the infant turns his head appropriately to the right, up and down, and as far left as the repertoire allows. Only if the repertoire is reduced to a single strategy is adaptive selection not possible.

Figure 4.5 shows the development of the adaptability of head movements in the norm population. At the age of three months, 80% of infants show adaptive head movements most of the time. At the age of five months, all infants have developed this ability.

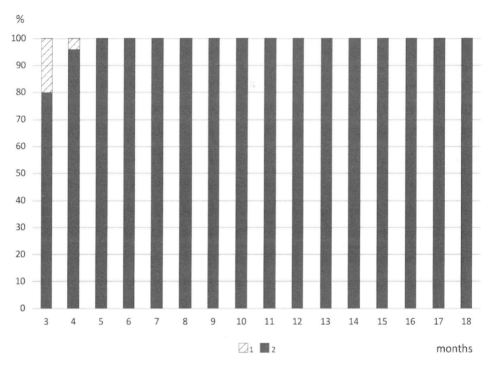

Figure 4.5 Development of adaptability of head movements in the norm population (item 3). Each bar represents 100 infants; infants who could not be assessed anymore while supine automatically got assigned score 2. The numbers in the legends denote the scores of the item.

4. *Posture of the head, presence of prevailing head position to one side (S)*

The presence of an asymmetry in prevailing head position is assessed. This item is assessed mainly on the basis of behaviour during the first three to five minutes of spontaneous, self-initiated movements. If the infant has a clear positional preference of the head to one side, after the first three to five minutes, the assessor uses an interesting object or her face to test whether the infant is able to move his head across the midline. The latter allows for the distinction between score 1 and score 2.

1 = strongly prevailing head position to the R/L
2 = moderately prevailing head position to the R/L
3 = no or mildly prevailing head position to one side

Score 1   Presence of an obligatory or virtually obligatory asymmetry in head position. The presentation of an attractive object and/or the examiner's face does not elicit head-turning movements across the midline to the contralateral side (Video 4.4). The prevailing side is recorded: R=right, L=left.

Score 2   Presence of a clear but not obligatory asymmetry in head position: that is, the head is turned more often to one side than to the other side. Score 2 implies that notwithstanding a prominently prevailing side position of the head, it is possible to elicit head movements across the midline when an attractive object and/or the face of the examiner is presented in that direction (Video 4.3). The prevailing side is recorded: R=right, L=left.

Score 3   The head is turned equally or almost equally often to the right and left side or is kept in the midline (Video 4.2). Infants with a minor oblique tilt of the head are also assigned score 3.

Figure 4.6 shows that at three months, 35% of the infants have a preferred head position to one side, mostly a moderately prevailing head position; only 3% have a strongly prevailing head position. With increasing age, the asymmetry in head position disappears and is absent at seven months.

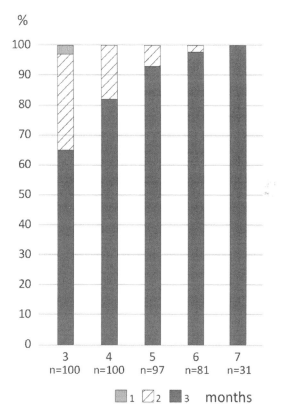

Figure 4.6 Development of asymmetry in head position while supine in the norm population (item 4). With increasing age fewer infants could be assessed in the supine position. The numbers in the legends denote the scores of the item.

5.   *Posture, presence of ATNR (V)*

The asymmetrical tonic neck reflex (ATNR) implies that head position induces reflex posturing of the limbs. More specifically, a sideways rotation of the head results in an increase of the tonus of the extensor muscles of the limbs at the facial side of the body and in a decrease of extensor tone on the contralateral side. This means that ATNR induces a 'fencing position' in which the arm on the side to which the face is turned extends and exorotates, and the arm at the other side flexes at the elbow and is raised at the shoulder (Magnus and de Kleijn 1912, Peiper 1963). A corresponding reaction in the legs may be observed. In this item, only ATNR posturing of the arms is taken into account. ATNR activity is present in typical individuals of any age, including adults (Aiello et al. 1988, Bruijn et al. 2013). However, typical brain function easily overrules the ATNR activity, allowing individuals with typical brain function to move their limbs independently of head position. The same holds true for infants: typically developing infants infrequently show ATNR postures. The presence of frequent or obligatory (i.e., stereotyped) ATNR posturing indicates the presence of brain dysfunction (Peiper 1963).

Note that this item assesses ATNR occurring during spontaneous, self-initiated movements, not its presence during interaction with the assessor and during object presentation.

    1 = frequently or obligatory occurring ATNR
    2 = no ATNR or occasional non-obligatory ATNR

Score 1   The infant frequently or obligatorily shows ATNR posturing of the arms (Figure 4.7).
Score 2   The infant does not or only rarely show ATNR posturing of the arms.

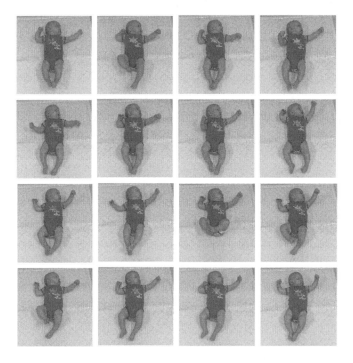

Figure 4.7 Frequently occurring ATNR on the left side in a three-month-old infant (item 5)

6. *Posture, presence of hyperextension of neck and trunk (V)*

Hyperextension of neck and trunk is described as an increased extensor tone of neck and trunk resulting in hyperextension of the spine. This movement pattern is usually accompanied by retraction of the shoulders (Touwen and Hadders-Algra 1983). This behaviour is part of the clinically described phenomenon of 'transient dystonia' (Drillien 1972, de Vries and de Groot 2002). Note that this item assesses hyperextension of neck and trunk occurring during spontaneous, self-initiated movements, not its presence during interaction with the assessor and during object presentation.

1 = frequently occurring or persistent hyperextension
2 = no or infrequent hyperextension

Score 1   The infant frequently or persistently shows hyperextension of neck and trunk. This may be expressed as hyperextension of neck and trunk, but also as prolonged or frequent 'bridging': that is, hyperextension of the trunk to such an extent that the infant bears weight only with his shoulders/neck and feet while his trunk is lifted from the support surface (Figure 4.8).
Score 2   The infant does not show or infrequently shows hyperextension of the neck and trunk.

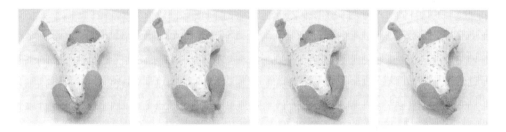

Figure 4.8 Hyperextension of neck and trunk in a three-month-old infant (item 6)

7. *Manipulative behaviour of hands and fingers (P)*

Manipulative behaviour of hands and fingers is spontaneously occurring goal-directed motor behaviour of hands and fingers, such as manipulation of clothes (e.g., the fingers of one or both hands repetitively touch, stroke, or grasp the onesie), playing with the hands in the midline (mutual manipulation of fingers; both hands are brought together in the midline, and the fingers of both hands repetitively touch, stroke, or grasp each other), and manual exploration of the knees, lower legs, or feet (Hopkins and Prechtl 1984). This item is based only on behaviour shown during the three to five minutes of spontaneous, self-initiated movements in the supine position and not during the part of the assessment when toys are presented.

The following actions are not regarded as manipulative behaviour of hands or fingers: (1) manipulative actions during rolling from the supine into the side position or the prone position; (2) a hand briefly touching the hair or the clothes without actual manipulation;

(3) scratching of the mattress; (4) sucking on thumb, finger, or hand. Yet hand play activity at or partly in the mouth is considered as manipulative activity.

> 1 = no manipulative behaviour
> 2 = manipulates clothes with hands in midline, on knees or feet or plays with hand(s) at mouth

Score 1   The infant does not manipulate with one or two hands and fingers. Sucking on a hand or finger may be present.
Score 2   The infant manipulates with one or two hands and fingers: for example, the infant manipulates his clothes or plays with his hands in the midline or at the mouth, or the infant's hand or hands exploratorily touch knees, lower legs, or feet (Video 4.5). This implies that a score 2 is also assigned when the infant manipulates with one hand only.

Figure 4.9 shows the development of manipulative behaviour of hands and fingers in the norm population. At three months, half the infants show manipulative behaviour in the supine position. This proportion gradually increases with age, so that at six months, 80% of infants exhibit manipulative behaviour.

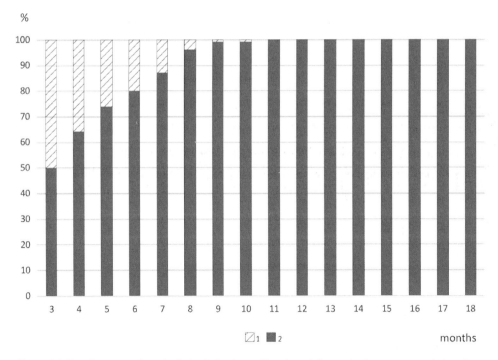

Figure 4.9 Development of manipulative behaviour of hands and fingers in the norm population (item 7). Each bar represents 100 infants; infants who could not be assessed anymore while supine automatically got assigned score 2. The numbers in the legends denote the scores of the item.

8. Variation in arm movements (V)

The size of the repertoire of movements of both arms during spontaneous, self-initiated movements is assessed. This implies that the presence of a typical movement repertoire in one arm in combination with a limited repertoire in the other arm results in the classification 'insufficient variation'. Note that this item assesses only motor behaviour occurring during spontaneous, self-initiated movements, not the variation in arm movements during interaction with the assessor and during object presentation.

    1 = insufficient variation
    2 = sufficient variation

Score 1   The infant shows a limited repertoire of arm movements in a limited number of directions, in a limited number of combinations of movements in the various joints and with limited variation over time. This means that specific stereotyped movement patterns persist or frequently occur. Examples of stereotyped patterns are extension–abduction movements or postures; flexion–adduction postures; and stereotyped, circular wrist movements (Figure 4.10; Video 4.6).

Score 2   The infant shows various movements of both arms in various directions (e.g., abduction and adduction movements, ante- and retroflexion movements, flexion, extension, rotation) and in various combinations of the three arm joints (shoulder, elbow, wrist) and two arms (Figure 4.10; Video 4.6).

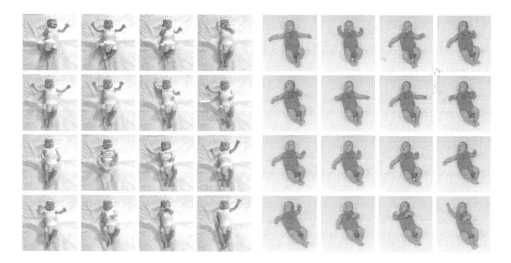

Figure 4.10 Spontaneous movements while supine of two four-month-old infants: quality of arm and finger movements (items 8 and 9). Left panel: sufficient variation in arm and finger movements; right panel: insufficient variation in arm and finger movements.

9.   Variation in finger movements (V)

The size of the repertoire of finger movements of both hands during spontaneous, self-initiated movements is assessed. This implies that the presence of a typical movement repertoire in one hand in combination with a limited repertoire in the other hand results in the classification 'insufficient variation'. Note that this item assesses only motor behaviour occurring during spontaneous, self-initiated movements, not the variation in finger movements during interaction with the assessor and during object presentation.

> 1 = insufficient variation
> 2 = sufficient variation

Score 1   The infant shows a limited repertoire of movements of fingers in a limited number of directions and in a limited number of combinations of movements of the individual fingers. For instance, frequently occurring fisting of the hands is denoted as insufficient variation (Figure 4.10; Video 4.6).

Score 2   The infant shows movements of the fingers in various directions and in various combinations of flexion, extension, abduction, and adduction of the two hands (Figure 4.10; Video 4.6).

10.   Tilting of pelvis (P)

Tilting of the pelvis is the movement in which the hips are flexed and moved slightly upwards. Depending on the degree to which the pelvis is tilted, hand-knee or hand-feet contact is possible (Hopkins and Prechtl 1984, Piper and Darrah 1994). Only pelvic movements during spontaneous, self-initiated movements are taken into account, not the pelvic movements during toy presentation.

> 1 = no tilting of pelvis
> 2 = tilts pelvis, but not in such a way that hands may touch the knees
> 3 = tilts pelvis in such a way that hands may touch the knees
> 4 = hands play with feet

Score 1   The infant does not tilt his pelvis in the supine position (Figure 4.11A).

Score 2   The infant tilts his pelvis to a limited extent: that is, he does not tilt it to such an extent that his hands may reach and touch his knees (Figure 4.11B).

Score 3   The infant tilts his pelvis in such a way that his hands may reach his knees. The hips are abducted and externally rotated, and the knees are flexed; if the infant moves the arms downwards to the knees, he may touch the knees. Actual touching of the knees, however, is not a prerequisite for score 3 as the focus of this item is on the degree of pelvic tilt (Figure 4.11C). A score 3 is not given in case of limited pelvic tilt in combination with strong anteflexion of the neck and shoulders, which, theoretically, also might result in touching of the knees. In that case, score 2 is assigned. Score 3 is also not assigned to an infant who barely tilts his pelvis but moves his knees in a frog-like position across the support surface in the direction of his hands. His score depends on the degree of pelvic tilt, resulting in either a 1 or a 2.

Score 4   The infant tilts his pelvis in such a way that his hands may manipulate his feet. The hips are flexed, the knees are semi-flexed or extended, the legs are lifted, and the feet are brought to the hands (Figure 4.11D). To obtain score 4, at least one hand should touch one foot. Manipulation of the feet may result in putting the toes into the mouth.

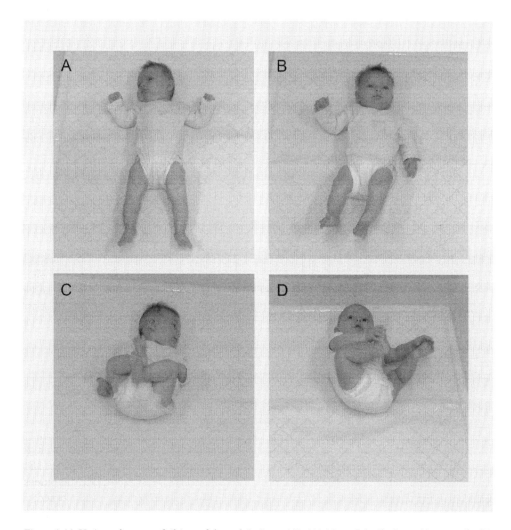

Figure 4.11 Various degrees of tilting of the pelvis (item 10). (A) No pelvis tilt (item 10: score 1); (B) minor pelvis tilt (item 10: score 2); (C) pelvis tilted so far that hands may touch the knees (item 10: score 3); (D) hands play with feet (item 10: score 4).

In case of asymmetrical performance, the performance of the best side is assigned.

Figure 4.12 shows the development of the tilting of the pelvis in the norm population. At three months, more than 80% of infants obtain score 3 ('tilts pelvis in such a way that hands may touch the knees'). With increasing age, an increased proportion of infants play

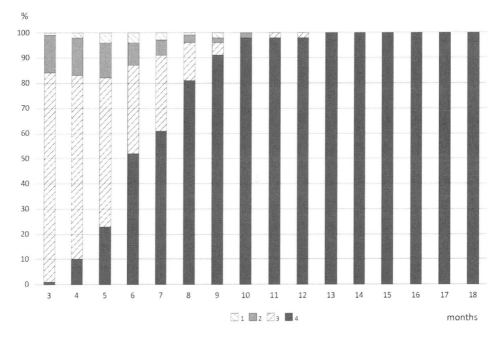

Figure 4.12 Development of tilting of the pelvis in the norm population (item 10). Each bar represents 100 infants; infants who could not be assessed anymore while supine automatically got assigned score 4. The numbers in the legends denote the scores of the item.

with the feet: 10% of the four-month-olds and 61% of the seven-month-olds. A minority of infants do not show pelvic tilt in the supine position (1% to 4%).

11.   Variation in leg movements (V)

The size of the repertoire of movements of both legs during spontaneous, self-initiated movements is assessed. This implies that the presence of a typical movement repertoire in one leg in combination with a limited repertoire in the other leg results in the classification 'insufficient variation'. Note that this item assesses only motor behaviour occurring during spontaneous, self-initiated movements, not the variation in leg movements during interaction with the assessor and during object presentation.

> 1 = insufficient variation
> 2 = sufficient variation

Score 1   The infant shows a limited repertoire of leg movements in a limited number of directions and in a limited number of movement combinations of the participating parts of the legs (Figure 4.13; Video 4.7). The presence of repetitive, stereotyped, circular ankle movements is also regarded as an expression of insufficient variation.

Score 2   The infant shows leg movements in various directions (e.g., flexion, extension, rotation, abduction, and adduction movements) and in various combinations of the three leg joints (hip, knee, ankle) and two legs (Figure 4.13; Video 4.7).

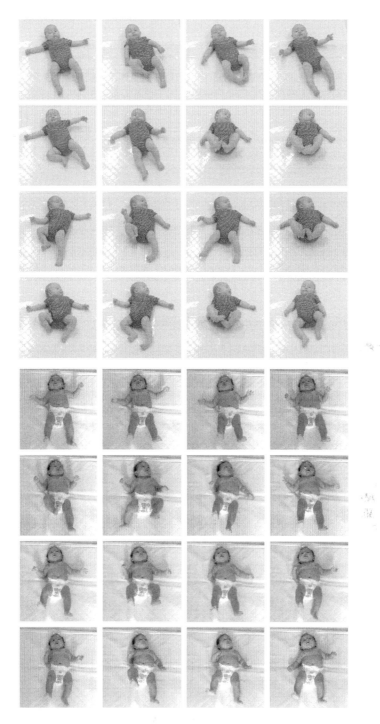

Figure 4.13 Spontaneous movements while supine of two three-month-old infants: quality of leg and toe movements (items 11 and 12). Top panel: sufficient variation in leg and toe movements; bottom panel: insufficient variation in leg and toe movements.

12.   *Variation in toe movements (V)*

The size of the repertoire of toe movements of both feet during spontaneous, self-initiated movements is assessed. This implies that the presence of a typical movement repertoire in one foot in combination with a limited repertoire in the other foot results in the classification 'insufficient variation'. Note that this item assesses only motor behaviour occurring during spontaneous, self-initiated movements, not the variation in toe movements during interaction with the assessor and during object presentation.

> 1 = insufficient variation
> 2 = sufficient variation

Score 1   The infant shows a limited repertoire of the movements of the toes: that is, movements in a limited number of directions. For instance, frequently occurring clawing of the toes or a consistent marked dorsiflexion of the big toe is denoted as insufficient variation (Figure 4.13; Video 4.7).

Score 2   The infant shows movements of the toes in various directions: for example, flexion, extension, abduction, and adduction of the toes of both feet (Figure 4.13; Video 4.7).

13.   *Rolling from the supine into the prone position (P)*

The infant's ability to roll from the supine into the prone position over the left and the right side is assessed. Rolling behaviour may be elicited by the presentation of toys. (See the procedure section in the introduction of this chapter.)

> 1 = no turning or rolling attempts
> 2 = makes 'wiggling' movements with the pelvis, but does not roll to side
> 3 = rolls to side, unilaterally R/L
> 4 = rolls to side, bilaterally
> 5 = turns unilaterally into prone R/L
> 6 = turns bilaterally into prone

Score 1   The infant does not show 'wiggling' movements or rolling to side or prone.

Score 2   The infant does not roll to a side position or into prone but makes 'wiggling' movements with the pelvis. Wiggling movements of the pelvis consist of small, irregular, undulating movements of the pelvis. These movements induce some tilting of the pelvis into sideways directions, but they do not result in rolling movements of the entire body into a side position (Video 4.8).

Score 3   The infant rolls unilaterally from supine to one side position (Video 4.8). The infant does not roll into prone position. To obtain score 3, the infant has to roll with his whole body to 90 degrees out of the supine position. The side to which the infant rolls is recorded: R=right and L=left.

Score 4   The infant rolls from supine to the left side and from supine to the right side position. The infant does not roll into prone.

Score 5   The infant turns unilaterally from supine into prone (Video 4.8). The side over which the infant turns is recorded: R=right and L=left.

Score 6   The infant turns bilaterally (i.e., over the left and over the right side) from supine into prone.

Figure 4.14 shows the development of rolling from the supine into the prone position in the norm population. At three months, about half the infants makes 'wiggling' movements of the pelvis, but they do not roll into side or prone position. At four months, about a quarter of the infants are able to roll into side or prone position, with 6% of them achieving prone position. Thereafter, the proportion of infants able to turn into the prone position rapidly increases from 25% at five months to 93% at nine months.

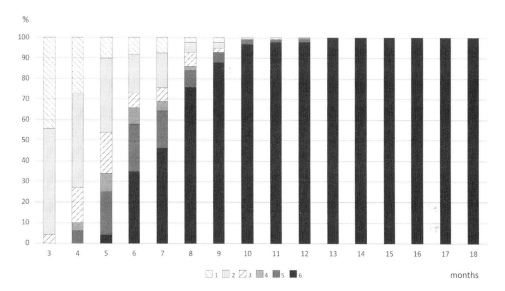

Figure 4.14 Development of rolling from supine into prone in the norm population (item 13). Each bar represents 100 infants; infants who could not be assessed anymore while supine automatically got assigned score 6. The numbers in the legends denote the scores of the item.

Reaching, grasping, and manipulation: additional information on testing procedures

The infant's ability to reach, grasp, and manipulate objects in the supine position is assessed. To this end, relatively small, attractive objects (Figure 4.2) are presented at arm's-length distance at various positions in space and a few times somewhat closer to the infant's body. (See the procedure section in the introduction of this chapter.) First, one toy is presented to the infant. For infants with emerging reaching and grasping abilities, present the toy in the midline at arm's-length distance and keep it there for a while. Arm's-length distance means not too far away and not too close to the body of the infant: for instance, not so close that an infant who produces prereaching movements directed towards the other hand in the midline might accidentally hit and grasp the toy. Pay close attention to the infant's visual attention. Repeat the toy presentation multiple times. When the infant is able to grasp the toy, allow him some time to manipulate the object. Next, the assessor retrieves the toy, and a second toy is presented. Again, the infant is given ample time to find his own solution to get it. If the infant is able to handle two objects, the infant is offered two objects in succession (not simultaneously!) several times. Thereafter, the assessor evaluates whether the infant is able to grasp an additional third object while holding two other ones. The latter means that the infant is able to hold two objects in one hand, implying that the infant is able to use the hand simultaneously as storage and a manipulative tool (Touwen 1976). Note that objects held in the mouth or objects held between hand and body are not considered 'objects held'.

When the assessor has determined how many objects the infant can handle at a time (performance item 14), the focus of the assessment shifts to the evaluation of variation and adaptability of arms and hands. To this end, the toys are presented one by one at a distance of about the length of the infant's arm (and not beyond!) at various positions in space. Several times, the object is also placed more closely to the infant's body. The spatial variation is needed to assess the infant's repertoire of arm and hand movements (variation) and ability to adapt reaching movements to the specifics of the condition (adaptability). To assess variation and adaptability of hand and finger movements, a variety of toys with different shapes and sizes is used. First, simple rings are presented, followed by the presentation of more complex objects, such as small puppets.

The reaching, grasping and manipulative abilities of both arms and hands are evaluated. In case of an asymmetry in arm-hand performance, the severity of the asymmetry is evaluated by also presenting toys on the side of the worst performing arm and hand. The performance of reaching and grasping is based on the best performance observed; in case of asymmetric arm movements, this is based on the performance of the best arm and hand. Note that the asymmetry itself is scored at item 15.

14.   *Reaching, grasping, and manipulation of objects (P)*

The infant's ability to reach, grasp, and manipulate objects in the supine position is assessed. The infant receives the score of the best performance, also when achieved with only one hand.

> 1 = does not reach and does not show prereaching movements
> 2 = does not reach but shows prereaching movements
> 3 = reaches towards object but does not grasp it
> 4 = reaches towards, grasps, and holds object but does not manipulate object
> 5 = reaches towards, holds, and manipulates 1 object
> 6 = reaches towards, holds, and manipulates 2 objects
> 7 = reaches towards and holds ≥3 objects

Score 1   The infant does not reach towards the object and does not show prereaching movements (see score 2).

Score 2   The infant does not reach towards the object but shows prereaching movements. Prereaching movements are movements of arms, hands and fingers in reaction to the presentation of an attractive object that do not result in an actual approach of the object (Trevarthen 1984, Hadders-Algra 2018c). Examples of prereaching movements are mutual manipulation of hands, hand-mouth contact movements, and flapping abduction movements of the arms in response to the presentation of an attractive object (Video 4.9). To distinguish between spontaneous arm movements that are not related to the object presentation (score 1) and prereaching, close attention is paid to the infant's visual attention. Prereaching is associated with clear visual fixation of the object, which often is accompanied by a facial expression of vivid interest and movements of the mouth. In spontaneous, non-goal-directed movements of the arms, the infant does not pay visual attention to the object.

Score 3 The infant reaches towards the object, gets close to it, but does not grasp it. Reaching is defined as making a goal-directed movement with one or both arms towards the object (Touwen 1976). The hand may or may not touch the object.

Score 4 The infant reaches towards, grasps, and holds the object. He does not manipulate the object within or between the hands, does not transfer the object from one hand to the other hand, and does not put the object into his mouth. Grasping is defined as approaching the object via a self-generated reaching movement with one or both hands, touching it, and getting hold of it. After grasping the object, the infant must hold the object for at least a few seconds to pass the item (Video 4.9). Note that the infant should grasp the object itself and that the object should not be put or pushed into the infant's hand by the examiner.

Score 5 The infant reaches towards, grasps, holds, and manipulates one object. Manipulation may consist, for example, of transferring the object to the other hand, moving the object within the hand, or putting the object into the mouth (Video 4.9). Infants who are able to grasp and hold two objects but who do not manipulate either object at all also are assigned score 5 (and not score 6).

Score 6 The infant holds one object and reaches towards a second object. This results in grasping of the second object, holding of the two objects, and some manipulation of at least one of the objects (Video 4.9). This also implies that infants who grasp a second object but immediately thereafter drop one of the objects are not assigned score 6.

Score 7 The infant holds two objects and reaches towards a third object. This results in grasping of the third object and holding of the three objects (Video 4.9). Manipulation is not required to obtain score 7; the focus of the item is on the ability to grasp an object with the hand that already holds another object. However, infants who grasp a third object but immediately thereafter drop one of the objects are not assigned score 7. Score 7 is also given when an infant is able to hold more than three objects.

Figure 4.15 shows the development of reaching, grasping, and manipulation while supine in the norm population. At three months, 20% of infants do not show reaching attempts, 50% show prereaching movements, and 7% are able to grasp at least one object. At four months, more than half of infants are able to grasp and manipulate at least one object, whereas at five months, 84% of infants have achieved this ability, with about 40% being able to grasp and manipulate two objects. At six months, the majority of infants are able to grasp and manipulate two objects. After the age of six months, the proportion of infants who can be assessed in the supine position rapidly drops.

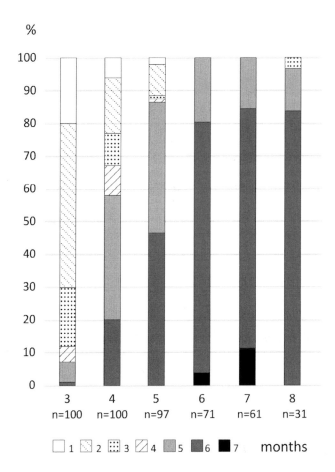

Figure 4.15 Development of reaching, grasping, and manipulation while supine in the norm population (item 14). With increasing age fewer infants could be assessed in the supine position. The numbers in the legends denote the scores of the item.

15.   *Reaching, grasping, and manipulating objects: presence of asymmetry (S)*

The presence of asymmetry in arm and hand movements during (pre)reaching, grasping, and manipulation is assessed.

0 = the infant does not show prereaching or reaching movements (item 14, score 1)

1 = strong asymmetry, R/L worst side
2 = moderate asymmetry, R/L worst side
3 = no or mild asymmetry

Score 0   The infant does not show prereaching or reaching movements; the infant received score 1 at item 14. Therefore, the item cannot be assessed. Note that score 0 does not imply a worse score than score 1, 2, or 3; it simply denotes that the score is not taken into account in the calculation of IMP scores.

Score 1   A marked difference between right and left side is present in the posture and movements of the arm and/or hand during (pre)reaching, grasping, and manipulation. This means that the arm and hand on one side of the body show a stereotypy and only exceptionally show other postures or movements: R=right and L=left (Video 4.10).

Score 2   The infant shows a moderate asymmetry in his posture and movements of arm and/or hand during (pre)reaching, grasping, and manipulation, but both sides are involved in the goal-directed activities of arms and hands: R=right and L=left (Video 4.10).

Score 3   The infant shows no or only a mild asymmetry in his posture and movements of the hand or arm during (pre)reaching, grasping, and manipulation of objects. This means that a mild hand preference may be present (Videos 4.10).

16.   *Variation in reaching movements of the arms (V)*

The size of the repertoire of movements of both arms is assessed. This implies that the presence of a typical movement repertoire in one arm in combination with a limited repertoire in the other arm results in the classification 'insufficient variation'. If an infant shows a mix of reaching and prereaching movements, both reaches and prereaches are taken into account. Also, the repertoire of arm movements between the various reaching movements is taken into account in the evaluation of the variation in arm movements during the assessment of reaching. The repertoire of arm movements is not assessed when the infant only shows prereaching movements.

0 = the infant does not show reaching movements (item 14: score 1 or 2)

1 = insufficient variation
2 = sufficient variation

Score 0   The infant does not show reaching movements; the infant received score 1 or score 2 at item 14. Therefore, the item cannot be assessed. Note that score 0 does not imply a worse score than score 1 or 2; it simply denotes that the score is not taken into account in the calculation of IMP scores.

Score 1   The infant shows a limited repertoire of reaching movements. The arm movements consist of a limited number of combinations of movements in shoulder, elbow, and wrist (Figure 4.16). Examples of stereotyped patterns are simple extension movements, unilateral stereotyped flexion posturing, and stereotyped flapping or rotatory wrist movements occurring between the reaches (Video 4.11).

Score 2   The infant shows reaching movements consisting of various combinations of movements in shoulder (abduction, adduction, flexion, extension, endorotation, and exorotation), elbow (flexion, extension, pronation, supination), and wrist (flexion, extension, adduction, abduction) of both arms (Figure 4.16, Video 4.11).

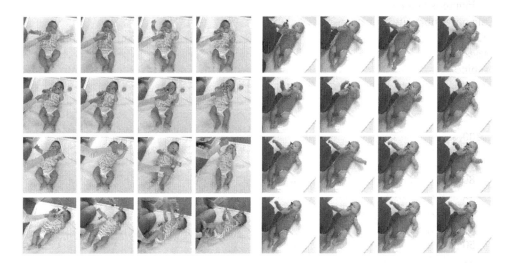

Figure 4.16 Variation in arm and hand movements during reaching, grasping, and manipulation while supine (items 16 and 18). Left panel: sufficient variation in arm and hand movements in boy of five months; right panel: insufficient variation in arm and hand movements in boy of four months.

17.   *Adaptability of reaching movements of the arms (A)*

Adaptability of reaching movements refers to the infant's ability to select in each situation the most appropriate and efficient reaching movement.

0 = the infant does not show reaching movements (item 14: score 1 or 2)

Majority of movements:

1 = no selection
2 = adaptive selection

Score 0   The infant does not show reaching movements, and therefore, the item cannot be assessed. If an infant only shows prereaching movements, score 0 is also assigned. In other words, score 0 is assigned to infants who received score 1 or 2 at item 14. Note that score 0 does not imply a worse score than score 1 or 2; it simply denotes that the score is not taken into account in the calculation of IMP scores.

Score 1   During the majority of reaching movements, the infant does not select a specific, efficient reaching strategy out of the repertoire of reaching arm movements for specific situations. Score 1 is also assigned to infants with a motor repertoire which is limited to one strategy (Video 4.12).

Score 2   During the majority of reaching movements, the infant selects specific and efficient reaching strategies out of the repertoire of reaching strategies: that is, strategies that suit situations best (Video 4.12). A prerequisite for adaptive selection is the presence of a repertoire that consists of more than one motor strategy.

Figure 4.17 shows the development of adaptability of arm movements while reaching in the norm population. Adaptability of arm movements while reaching emerges at five months: 12% of the infants who are able to reach mostly show adaptive movements of the arm. At seven months, 45% of the infants show adaptive movements of the arms while reaching in the supine position. After that age, increasingly fewer infants can be assessed while supine.

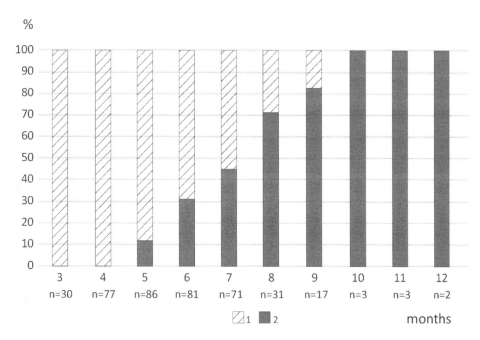

Figure 4.17 Development of adaptability of arm movements during reaching in the norm population (item 17). With increasing age fewer infants could be assessed in the supine position. The numbers in the legends denote the scores of the item.

18.   *Variation of hand movements while reaching, grasping, and manipulating (V)*

The size of the repertoire of movements of both hands is assessed. This implies that the presence of a typical movement repertoire in one hand in combination with a limited repertoire in the other hand results in the classification 'insufficient variation'. The repertoire of hand movements between the various reaching, grasping, and manipulative movements is also taken into account in the evaluation of the variation in hand movements during the assessment of reaching. The repertoire of hand movements is not assessed when the infant only shows prereaching movements.

0 = the infant does not show reaching movements (item 14: score 1 or 2)

1 = insufficient variation
2 = sufficient variation

Score 0   The infant does not show reaching movements, and therefore, the item cannot be assessed; the infant received score 1 or 2 at item 14. Note that score 0 does not imply a worse score than score 1 or 2; it simply denotes that the score is not taken into account in the calculation of IMP scores.

Score 1   The infant shows only a limited number of ways to move his hands while pre-reaching and reaching for, grasping, and manipulating objects. He shows a limited repertoire of hand and finger movements with little variation in the ways in which the finger movements and positions are combined. Examples of stereotyped movement patterns are hand opening-closing movements in which the fingers of the hand move more or less synchronously with few independent finger movements and a consistent unilateral fisting posture (Figure 4.16; Video 4.11).

Score 2   The infant shows various ways to move his hands during prereaching and reaching for, grasping, and manipulating objects. He shows variation in the ways in which the various possible finger movements and positions are combined (Figure 4.16; Video 4.11).

19. *Adaptability of hand movements while reaching, grasping, and manipulating (A)*

Adaptability of hand movements refers to the infant's ability to select the most appropriate hand and finger movements in each situation. Adaptability of hand movements can be assessed when the hand approaches the object ('is the hand preshaped to the form and size of the object?') and during actual grasping of the object and object manipulation.

0 = the infant does not show reaching movements (item 14: score 1 or 2)

Majority of movements:

1 = no selection
2 = adaptive selection

Score 0   The infant does not show reaching movements, and therefore, the item cannot be assessed; the infant received score 1 or 2 at item 14. Note that score 0 does not imply a worse score than score 1 or 2; it simply denotes that the score is not taken into account in the calculation of IMP scores.

Score 1   During the majority of reaching, grasping, and manipulative movements, the infant does not select a specific and efficient strategy out of his repertoire of grasping and/or manipulation strategies for specific situations (Video 4.12). Score 1 is also assigned to infants with a motor repertoire which is limited to one strategy.

Score 2   During the majority of reaching, grasping, and manipulative movements, the infant selects specific and efficient strategies out of his repertoire of grasping and/or manipulation strategies: that is, strategies that suit specific situations best. A prerequisite for adaptive selection is the presence of a repertoire that consists of more than one motor strategy.

20. *Tremor during prereaching and reaching (F)*

A tremor is an involuntary, oscillating movement with a fixed frequency (Piña-Garza and James 2019). Two types of tremors can be distinguished: the most frequently occurring type is a tremor with high frequency (≥ 6/sec) and low amplitude (≤ 3 cm). The other, less often observed type is a tremor with low frequency (<6/sec) and high amplitude (>3 cm) (Touwen 1976). At this item, tremors superimposed on reaching or prereaching movements are assessed. Note that irregular zig-zag movements are not regarded as tremor.

0 = the infant does not show prereaching or reaching movements (item 14: score 1)

1 = frequently present, describe type:
2 = not or occasionally present

Score 0   The infant does not show prereaching or reaching movements; the infant received score 1 at item 14. Therefore, the item cannot be assessed. Note that score 0 does not imply a worse score than score 1 or 2; it simply denotes that the score is not taken into account in the calculation of IMP scores.

Score 1   The infant shows tremors during the majority of prereaching, reaching, grasping, and manipulative movements (Video 4.13). Describe the type of tremor. The most commonly observed tremors are tremors with a high frequency (≥6/sec) and a low amplitude (≤3 cm) and those with a low frequency (<6/sec) and a high amplitude (>3 cm).
Score 2   The infant does not or only occasionally shows a tremor during prereaching, reaching, grasping, and manipulative movements. Tremor may be present during some of the prereaching, reaching, grasping, and manipulative movements, but during the majority of arm and hand movements, tremor is absent.

21.   Fluency of motor behaviour while supine (F)

Fluency of motor behaviour during the entire supine situation, including the reaching and grasping part, is assessed. Fluency of motor behaviour denotes the presence of smooth and graceful movements without effort. Fluency in particular points to the velocity profile of movements. Fluent movements are characterized by gradual accelerations and decelerations (Hadders-Algra 2004).

Majority of movements:

1 = non-fluent: stiff, jerky, floppy/sluggish, otherwise:
2 = fluent

Score 1   The majority of the movements are non-fluent, indicating that they are not smooth, supple, or graceful. Various sorts of non-fluency can be distinguished, and an infant may show different types of non-fluent movements during a single assessment (Video 4.14). Examples of non-fluent movements are stiff movements, jerky movements, and sluggish movements. Stiff movements lack ease of movement and give the impression of resistance. Jerky movements denote the presence of sudden, abrupt movements. Floppy or sluggish movements are limp, torpid, and slow. If the non-fluent character of the movements cannot be described as stiff, jerky, or floppy/sluggish, describe the non-fluency in alternative, more appropriate words
Score 2   The majority of the movements have a fluent character, indicating that the movements are smooth, supple, and graceful (Video 4.14).

5 Assessment of motor behaviour while prone

This chapter contains the description of the IMP items assessed in the prone position. Prone positions do not just include the situations in which the infant lies with his belly on the support surface; they also include locomotion while prone: for example, abdominal crawling or crawling on hands and knees. The prone position is evaluated in all infants; assessment in this position cannot be skipped. This also means that infants who bottom shuffle should be put into the prone position and that in infants who walk independently crawling should be assessed.

Procedure

Young infants are placed in the prone position with their heads in the midline, both shoulders in adduction, and both elbows in flexion, with the hands approximately in line with the ears. This means that the infant should not be propped into an elbow support position with the elbows in front of the shoulders, nor should the elbows be placed under the trunk. If the infant does not lift his head and does not turn his head to a side position after a few seconds, the examiner moves the infant's head into a side position. If the infant spontaneously turns his head with a minimal lift to one side and continues to lie with his head in a side position on the support surface, the assessor repositions the head in the midline after about one minute. If the infant thereafter does not lift or turn his head, the assessor turns the head of the infant to a side position. If, during placement into the prone position, the infant 'lands' on extended arms, the assessor repositions the arms and hands of the infant into the position just described: that is, with both shoulders in adduction and both elbows in flexion, with the hands approximately in line with the ears.

If the infant moves one or both arms from the initial starting position into a seemingly 'awkward' position, do not reposition the arm of the infant as this is part of the infant's spontaneous motor behaviour.

Older infants usually spontaneously adopt prone positions: they may roll from supine into prone, or they may move from sitting into prone. However, infants who have mastered the ability to walk independently may no longer adopt the prone position to play and move around. They may be playfully invited to perform activities in the prone position, which implies, in these infants, activities involving crawling behaviour.

In general, the infant's self-generated motor behaviour in the prone position is assessed for several minutes. In contrast to assessment in the supine position, the assessor may immediately start to interact with the infant in order to promote the self-generated movements of the infant. The minimum time needed for the assessment of the prone

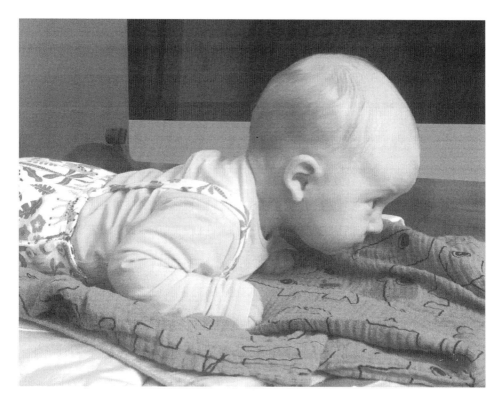

Figure 5.1 Starting position while prone in young infants: both shoulders are placed in adduction and both elbows in flexion with the hands approximately in line with the ears. The three-month-old infant could lift the head for some seconds, but did not maintain the head lift for ten seconds.

position items in infants who do not locomote while prone is one minute. In young infants and infants with neurological impairment, the duration of the prone assessment may be limited due to the infant's difficulties in lifting his head. As prolonged positioning in the prone position may be too stressful for these infants, it is better to assess prone behaviour by means of two or three stretches of 20 to 30 seconds in the prone position, which are alternated with periods in the supine position. In infants with limited capacity to lift their heads, head lifting may be promoted by positioning the assessor's or caregiver's face vis-a-vis the infant's head. Presentation of an adult person's face is more effective in attracting the young infant's interest than the presentation of a toy as infants have an innate preference for human faces (Johnson et al. 2015). The caregiver or the assessor verbally encourages the infant to look up.

Some infants remain in the prone position relatively briefly as bursts of hyperextension of the neck and trunk move them into the supine position. When this happens, the infant is returned to the prone position as often as needed to obtain sufficient time for the assessment of motor behaviour in that position.

For the evaluation of arm and hand movements in the prone position, toys are presented in various directions and at various distances on and above the support surface in front of the infant. Toys are also used to elicit progression in the prone position. The toys are presented laterally to elicit pivoting and in front to elicit forward progression. Suitable toys to elicit progression in the prone position are balls, cars, and trains (see Video 5.1).

As mentioned before, infants who have developed the ability to stand or walk, or who move around by means of bottom shuffling, also should be assessed in the prone position to assess motor behaviour in this position. This may be achieved by means of playing with a car or a ball. It certainly helps if the assessor or the caregiver also adopts the prone position and crawls around. Crawling behaviour may also be elicited by the presence of a piece of furniture (chair, table) that can serve as a tunnel. Usually, infants who walk independently only remain in the prone position for a short period, but the combination of various short periods will allow for the assessment of the prone items. The minimum amount of crawling behaviour needed to assess the prone items in crawling infants is two stretches of crawling, each consisting of at least four crawling 'steps' on hands and knees.

22.   Head lift in prone (P)

The infant's ability to lift his head and to produce head movements that allow him to look around is assessed with the help of the presentation of the examiner's or caregiver's face or the presentation of attractive toys.

> 1 = does not lift or turn head
> 2 = does turn head to side position with a minimal lift of the head
> 3 = lifts head for a few seconds but no longer
> 4 = maintains head lifted for at least ten seconds, but has some difficulty in looking around
> 5 = maintains head lifted and looks around

Score 1   The infant does not lift his head from the support surface and does not rotate the head into side position. If this happens, the examiner turns the infant's head into side position after a few seconds.

Score 2   The infant rotates his head into side position with an imperceptible lift of his head (see Video 5.2).

Score 3   The infant lifts his head for a few seconds but does not maintain his head lifted for at least ten seconds (Figure 5.1; see Video 5.2).

Score 4   The infant lifts his head and maintains his head lifted for at least ten seconds but has difficulty turning his head in all directions. Infants who are able to look around for at least ten seconds but also show sudden dropping movements of their heads also receive score 4 (see Video 5.2).

Score 5   The infant lifts his head, keeps it lifted, and easily turns his head in any direction (Figure 5.2; see Video 5.2).

Figure 5.3 shows the development of the head lift while prone in the norm population. At three months, 13% of the infants are not able to lift their heads for a few seconds,

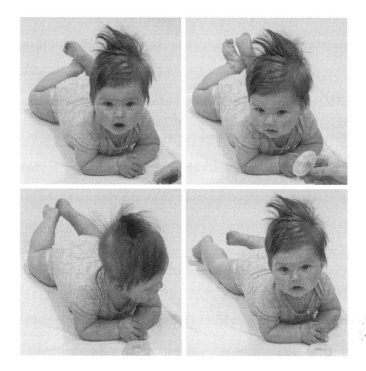

Figure 5.2 Head lift while prone in a six-month-old girl: she is able to lift the head more than ten seconds and easily turns the head in any direction (item 22)

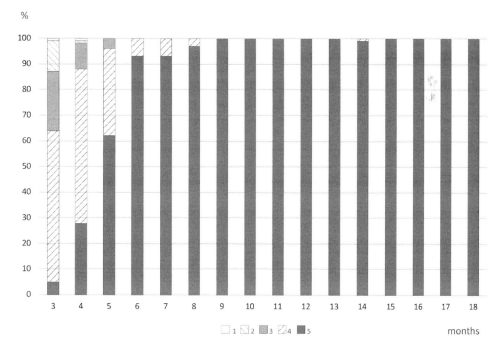

Figure 5.3 Development of head lift while prone in the norm population (item 22). Each bar represents 100 infants. The numbers in the legends denote the scores of the item.

whereas the majority (64%) are able to lift their heads for at least ten seconds. The ability to keep the head lifted and to look around easily rapidly increases from 5% at three months to 62% at five months to 93% at six months.

23.   *Position of the head, presence of prevailing head position to one side (S)*

The presence of an asymmetry in prevailing head position is assessed.

> 0 = the infant does not lift and rotate head into side position (item 22: score 1)
>
> 1 = strongly prevailing head position to the R/L
> 2 = moderately prevailing head position to the R/L
> 3 = no or mildly prevailing head position to one side

Score 0   The infant does not lift and rotate his head into side position; the head remains on the support surface; the infant received score 1 at item 22. When this happens, the examiner turns the infant's head into side position (see item 22). Note that score 0 does not imply a worse score than score 1, 2, or 3; it simply denotes that the score is not taken into account in the calculation of IMP scores.

Score 1   The infant keeps the head turned to one side during virtually all the time. The presentation of an interesting face or object does not elicit head turning movements across the midline to the contralateral side: R=right and L=left (Figure 5.4; see Video 5.3).

Score 2   The infant keeps his head turned substantially longer to one side than to the other side. Score 2 implies that, notwithstanding the dominance of the head to be turned into one direction, turning of the head across the midline can be elicited by presenting an interesting face or object in that direction: R=right and L=left (Video 5.3).

Score 3   The head is equally or almost equally often turned to the right and to the left side or is kept in the midline (Figure 5.2; see Video 5.3).

Figure 5.5 shows that at three months, 40% of the infants have a preferred head position to one side, including 12% having a strongly prevailing head position. With increasing age, the prevalence of asymmetric head position while prone rapidly decreases to 9% at five months and 0% at six months.

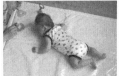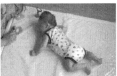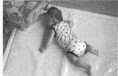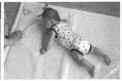

Figure 5.4 Infant of three months with strongly prevailing head position to the left while prone; the infant is not able to move the head across the midline (item 23)

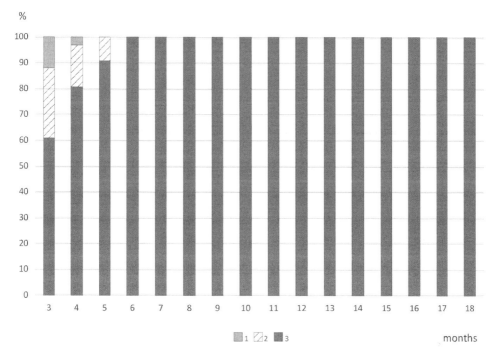

Figure 5.5 Asymmetry in head position while prone in the norm population (item 23). Each bar represents 100 infants. The numbers in the legends denote the scores of the item.

24. *Variation in head movements (V)*

The size of the repertoire of head movements is assessed.

    1 = insufficient variation
    2 = sufficient variation

Score 1   The infant shows a limited repertoire of head movements in a limited number of directions. An example is a head preference to one side with minimal ability to cross the midline. When the infant does not move his head, a score 1 is also assigned.

Score 2   The infant shows movements of his head in various directions: for example, to the right and to the left and anteflexion, retroflexion, and lateroflexion movements (Figure 5.2; see Video 5.1).

25. *Adaptability of head movements (A)*

Adaptability of head movements refers to the infant's ability to select the most appropriate and efficient head movement in each situation (see Video 5.4).
Majority of movements:

    1 = no adaptive selection
    2 = adaptive selection

Score 1   During the majority of movements, the infant does not select the most appropriate and efficient movement strategy out of his repertoire of head movements for the specific situation. The infant may explore various head movements but has difficulties moving his head efficiently in the desired direction. Score 1 is also assigned if the infant has a markedly reduced movement repertoire consisting of only one strategy.

Score 2   During the majority of movements, the infant is able to choose the most appropriate and efficient movement strategy out of his motor repertoire for the specific situations most of the time. For instance, the infant is able to turn his head promptly at the right moment to the right spot: for example, to an attractive object. Note that it is also possible to show adaptive motor behaviour when the movement repertoire (variation) is reduced. For instance, if an infant has a reduced motor repertoire, consisting of a limitation in turning his head to the left side, a score 2 is given if the infant turns his head appropriately to the right, up and down, and as far to the left as the repertoire allows. Adaptive selection is not possible only if the repertoire is reduced to a single strategy.

Figure 5.6 shows the development of adaptability of head movements while prone in the norm population. At three months, almost 30% of infants mostly show adaptive head movements in the prone position. The proportion of infants with adaptive head movements gradually increases so that at five months, 85% of infants achieve this ability, and at seven months, all infants do.

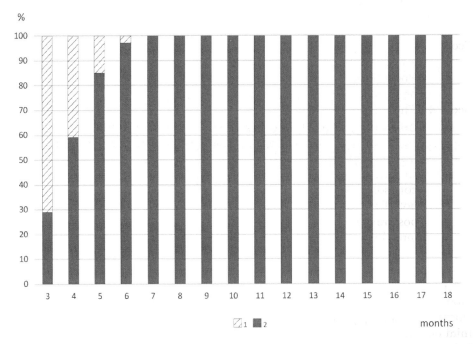

Figure 5.6 Development of adaptability of head movements while prone in the norm population (item 25). Each bar represents 100 infants. The numbers in the legends denote the scores of the item.

26.   *Functional ability of shoulder girdle while prone (P)*

The functional ability of the shoulder girdle while prone is the capacity of the infant to lift his head and the upper part of his thorax up by active use of arms and hands (Figure 5.7; Video 5.5).

> 1 = does not use arms and hands to move head and thorax up
> 2 = uses arms and hands to move head and thorax up but does not succeed in active elbow and lower arm support
> 3 = is supported by elbows and lower arms
> 4 = lifts upper part of thorax by 'standing' on hands and extended arms

Score 1   The infant does not use both arms and hands to move his head and thorax up. This implies that a score 1 is also assigned when both arms remain in the starting position imposed by the examiner: that is, with both shoulders in adduction and both elbows in flexion, with the hands approximately in line with the ears. In addition, score 1 is assigned to infants who lift their heads by means of neck extension or neck and trunk extension without using arm support.

Score 2   The infant uses both arms and hands to move his head and thorax up but does not succeed in active elbow and lower arm support (Figure 5.7A). The head and upper part of the thorax may be lifted for a few seconds, but they are not stabilized by elbow support. A swimming position in which the infant extends his back and spreads his arms to both sides may be present (Touwen 1976, Piper and Darrah 1994).

Score 3   The infant lifts his head and the upper part of his thorax up by active elbow and lower arm support of both arms (Figure 5.7B). The infant moves his elbows in line with or in front of his shoulders, and his weight is distributed on forearms, hands, and trunk (Piper and Darrah 1994).

Score 4   The infant lifts the upper part of his thorax up by 'standing' on one or two hands and extended arms. In this position, the elbow is somewhat in front of the shoulder, and the arm is more or less extended and bears weight (Piper and Darrah 1994). The angle between the supporting arm and the support surface is at least 45 degrees (Figure 5.7C). A movement consisting of a minimal lift of the elbow from the support surface does not allow for a score 4. Score 4 is also not assigned if the arm extension posture was imposed accidentally by the assessor when putting the infant into the prone position; it should be a movement initiated by the infant himself.

Figure 5.8 shows the development of the functional ability of the shoulder girdle while prone in the norm population. At three months, about half the infants try to achieve elbow and lower arm support but are not able to accomplish this, whereas about one-third do not use arms and hands to move the thorax up. At four months, 24% of the infants are able to achieve elbow and lower arm support; at five months, this rises to almost 60%. At six to seven months, about 95% of the infants are able to achieve elbow

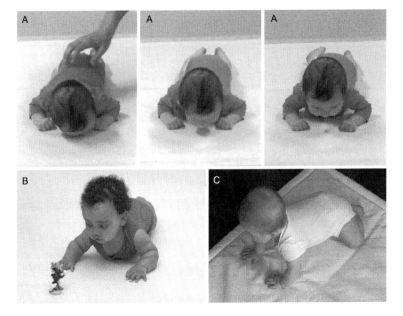

Figure 5.7 Functional ability of shoulder girdle while prone. (A) Uses arms and hands to move head and thorax up, but does not succeed in active elbow and lower arm support; (B) supported by elbows and lower arms; (C) 'stands' on hands and extended arms.

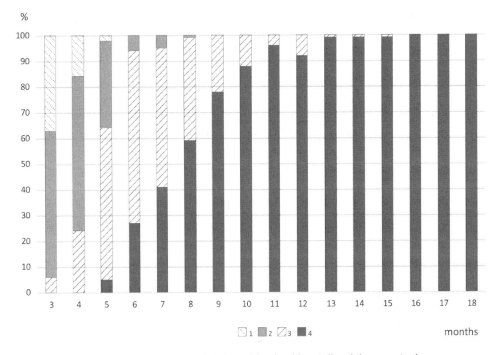

Figure 5.8 Development of the functional ability of the shoulder girdle while prone in the norm population (item 26). Each bar represents 100 infants. The numbers in the legends denote the scores of the item.

support or to 'stand' on hands and extended arms. The ability to 'stand' on hands and extended arms emerges at five months; at six months, about a quarter of the infants have acquired this skill, after which its prevalence gradually rises to more than 90% in infants aged 11 months and older.

27. *Functional ability of arms and hands while prone (P)*

To test the functional ability of the arms and hands while prone, arm and hand movements are elicited by presenting attractive toys on the support surface in front of the infant at immediate grasping distance. If the infant is able to grasp and manipulate one or more toys, additional toys are placed a bit farther away, at about arm's-length distance, on or somewhat above the support surface. The examiner does not put the toys into the infant's hands; the infant is challenged to get hold of them. If the infant is able to crawl on hands and knees, the examiner also tries to elicit reaching out for a toy (Video 5.6). This may be difficult in infants who are able to walk independently as they usually spent little time in the prone position: that is, when crawling.

1 = has difficulties using arms and hands for postural control and does not use hands for other activities
2 = uses one or two arms and hands for postural control and does not use hands for other activities
3 = uses one or two arms for postural control while hands show some play activity
4 = uses one arm for postural support and may use the contralateral arm and hand for reaching and manipulation

Score 1   The infant has difficulties using his arms and hands for postural control and does not use his hands for other activities. Score 1 or 2 at item 26 implies score 1 here (Figure 5.7A).
Score 2   The infant uses one or two arms and hands for postural control; he does not use his hands for other activities such as reaching, grasping, or manipulation of toys (Figure 5.9A).
Score 3   The infant uses one or two arms for postural control and shows some play activities of his hands. The infant does grasp and/or manipulate nearby toys but does not reach out for toys at arm's-length distance (Figure 5.9B).
Score 4   The infant uses one arm only for postural support and lifts and uses the other arm and hand for reaching, grasping, and manipulation. The infant gets hold of nearby toys and toys placed at arm's-length distance (Figure 5.9C). The hand of the supporting arm may or may not be involved in the manipulative activities. Score 4 is also assigned to infants who crawl around on hands and knees but do not stop to play in this position. Score 4 is not assigned to infants who achieve a swimming posture and get hold of an object without using arm support; these infants are assigned a score 1, 2, or 3, depending on their overall performance while prone.

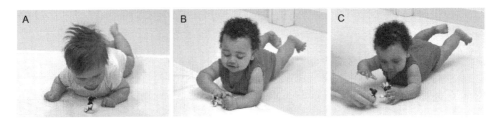

Figure 5.9 Functional ability of arms and hands while prone (item 27). (A) Uses one or two arms and hands for postural control, and does not use hands for other activities; (B) uses one or two arms for postural control while hands show some play activity; (C) uses one arm for postural support and uses contralateral arm and hand for reaching and manipulation.

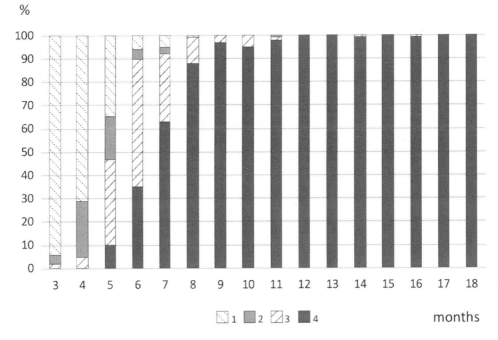

Figure 5.10 Development of the functional ability of arms and hands while prone in the norm population (item 27). Each bar represents 100 infants. The numbers in the legends denote the scores of the item.

Figure 5.10 shows the development of the functional ability of the arms and hands in the prone position in the norm population. The ability to use the hands while prone for play activity is present in a few infants aged three to four months. By the age of five months, about half the infants can play with their hands while prone. At six months, 90% of infants use their hands for play while prone, with about one-third of them being able to do so while being supported by only one arm. The latter ability (i.e., being able to use one arm for postural support and the other for reaching, grasping, and manipulation) increases further to more than 60% at seven months and more than 90% from nine months onwards.

28. Posture and movements of arms and hands during activity while prone: presence of asymmetry (S)

The presence of asymmetry in posture and movements of the arms and hands in prone is assessed. Special attention is paid to the presence of mild or marked stereotypes in motor behaviour of one upper extremity (Video 5.7).

0 = both arms remain in position imposed by examiner (item 26: score 1)

1 = strong asymmetry, R/L worst side
2 = moderate asymmetry, R/L worst side
3 = no or mild asymmetry

Score 0   Both arms remain in the starting position imposed by the examiner; the infant received score 1 at item 26. Note that score 0 does not imply a worse score than score 1, 2, or 3; it simply denotes that the score is not taken into account in the calculation of IMP scores.

Score 1   One upper extremity shows a clear stereotypy while prone while the other upper extremity does not. For example, the arm is held in stereotyped shoulder adduction and elbow flexion, and the hand is fisted; the arm and hand do not or only exceptionally show other postures and movements: R=right and L=left.

Score 2   One upper extremity shows a moderate stereotypy while prone while the other upper extremity does not. The moderate stereotypy may consist of, for example, a frequently occurring flexion of the arm with the hand held in fist or a frequently occurring abduction of the shoulder with extension of the elbow. Yet the affected extremity also shows some other arm and hand postures and movements: R=right and L=left.

Score 3   Both arms and hands contribute equally or almost equally to postural control and goal-directed movements while prone, and both arms and hands show more or less the same strategy or strategies.

29. Progression while prone: development of crawling (P)

The infant is encouraged to displace himself while in the prone position by placing attractive toys at some distance from the infant (Video 5.1). The toys may be placed sideways to elicit pivoting or in front of the infant to elicit forward movements. For infants with limited abilities to move forward, the toys are placed just out of arm's reach. Older infants may be challenged to move forward by rolling a ball or moving a toy car or train. The most advanced way of progression while prone shown by the infant is recorded. (See also the procedures in the chapter's introduction; Video 5.8.)

1 = does not show pivoting or crawling while prone
2 = pivoting
3 = abdominal crawling, uses arms and/or legs
4 = crawls on hands and knees, abdomen free from support surface

Score 1   The infant does not show pivoting or crawling while prone. Usually, the infant does show leg movements, but these movements are not associated with evident displacement of the infant. Infants with bursts of hyperextension of the neck and trunk who do not show progression while prone are also assigned score 1. In addition, infants who use bottom shuffling as the only way to move around (i.e., when they do not displace their body in prone the position) are assigned score 1.

Score 2   Pivoting movements consist of movements of trunk, arms, and legs that result in spatial displacement around the centre of the body: that is, around a vertical axis through the umbilicus (Largo et al. 1985). In order to achieve score 2, spatial displacement should be more than 30 degrees (Figure 5.11A).

Score 3   The infant shows abdominal crawling with use of arms and/or legs. This means that forward progression of at least 10 centimetres while prone is achieved by means of arm and/or leg movements while the abdomen remains in contact with the support surface. The movements of the arms and legs may or may not be co-ordinated (Figure 5.11B).

Score 4   The infant shows a variant of crawling in which arms and legs are used for propulsion while the abdomen is free from the support surface (Figure 5.11C). The most commonly observed form is crawling on hands and knees; in order to meet the criterion for score 4, the infant needs to produce at least four alternating leg movements ('steps') on his knees. But alternative forms may also be observed, such as 'bear' crawling, during which the infant crawls on hands and feet (Figure 5.11D), and bunny-hopping (a form of prone locomotion in which the infant 'jumps' forward by a sudden extension movement of the hips) (McGraw 1943, Largo et al. 1985, Bottos et al. 1989, Adolph et al. 1998).

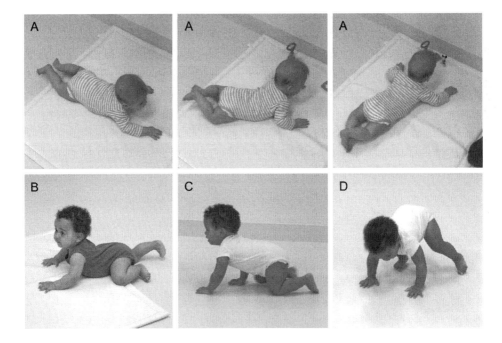

Figure 5.11 Progression while prone (item 29). (A) Pivoting; (B) abdominal crawling; (C) crawls on all fours; (D) bear crawling.

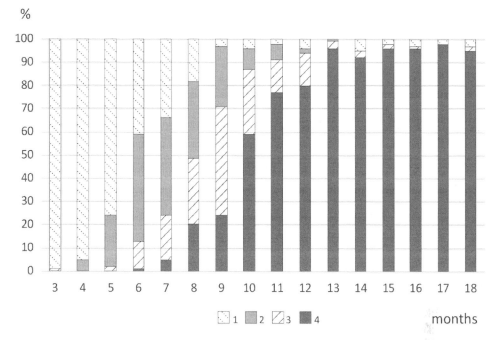

Figure 5.12 Development of progression while prone, i.e., development of crawling in the norm population (item 29). Each bar represents 100 infants. The numbers in the legends denote the scores of the item.

Figure 5.12 shows the development of progression while prone (i.e., the development of crawling) in the norm population. Below the age of five months, few infants displace themselves in the prone position. At five months, 22% of the infants pivot, and at six and seven months, some 40% of the infants use this method to displace themselves while prone. Abdominal crawling emerges at five months; it is used by 12% of the infants at six months, becoming the most prevalent way to locomote while prone (47%) at nine months. Crawling on hands and knees emerges at six months, and at ten months, about 60% of infants move around in this way. From 13 months onwards, crawling on hands and knees occurs in more than 90% of infants.

30. Variation in pre-crawling movements of the legs (V)

Pre-crawling movements are movements of the legs in the prone position which do not result in progression. Pre-crawling movements also include the leg movements produced during pivoting and those that result in some caudal displacement.

The size of the movement repertoire of both legs is assessed (Video 5.9). This implies that the presence of a typical movement repertoire in one leg in combination with a limited repertoire in the other leg results in the classification 'insufficient variation'.

0 = shows progression while prone (item 29: score 3 or 4)

1 = insufficient variation
2 = sufficient variation

Score 0   The infant shows progression while prone; the infant received score 3 or 4 at item 29. Note that score 0 does not imply a worse score than score 1 or 2; it simply denotes that the score is not taken into account in the calculation of IMP scores.

Score 1   The infant shows only a limited repertoire of leg movements in a limited number of directions in a limited number of movement combinations of the participating parts of the legs. Score 1 is also given to infants who remain immobile while prone. An example is the presence of simple flexion-extension movements of the legs without differentiated ankle movements.

Score 2   The infant shows leg movements in various directions (e.g., flexion, extension, rotation, abduction, and adduction) and in various combinations of the three leg joints (hip, knee, ankle) and two legs.

31. Rolling from prone into supine (P)

If the infant has not shown rolling movements during the first few minutes while prone, the ability of the infant to turn over into supine is elicited by presenting attractive toys in the two rolling directions. The toys are presented just out of reach of the infant in the arm area between 90 and 180 degrees of shoulder abduction.

The way in which the infant achieves the turning movement is not taken into account as we experienced that the distinction between 'atypical' rolling (e.g., with hyperextension of neck and trunk) and 'typical' rolling could not be assessed reliably.

0 = does not show rolling, as the infant prefers to change position in space by means of crawling (item 29: scores 3 or 4), bottom shuffling, or walking.

1 = no turning or rolling attempts while not able to sit or crawl
2 = rolls to side unilaterally R/L
3 = rolls to side bilaterally
4 = turns unilaterally into supine R/L
5 = turns bilaterally into supine

Score 0   The infant does not show rolling because he has the ability to sit, crawl, or walk. Crawling means the presence of abdominal crawling or crawling with the abdomen free from the support surface (item 29: scores 3 or 4). Note that score 0 does not imply a worse score than scores 1 to 4; it simply denotes that the score is not taken into account in the calculation of IMP scores.

Score 1   The infant does not show turning or rolling attempts and is not able to sit, crawl, or walk.
Score 2   The infant rolls unilaterally from prone to side position. The rolling does not result in supine position. The side to which the infant rolls is recorded: R=right and L=left.
Score 3   The infant rolls from prone to left side and from prone to the right side position. The turning does not result in supine position.
Score 4   The infant turns unilaterally from prone into supine (Figure 5.13). The side over which the infant turns is recorded: R=right and L=left.
Score 5   The infant turns bilaterally (i.e., over the left and over the right side) from prone into supine.

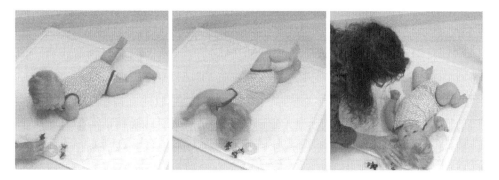

Figure 5.13 Infant of five months rolls over the left side from prone into supine position (item 31)

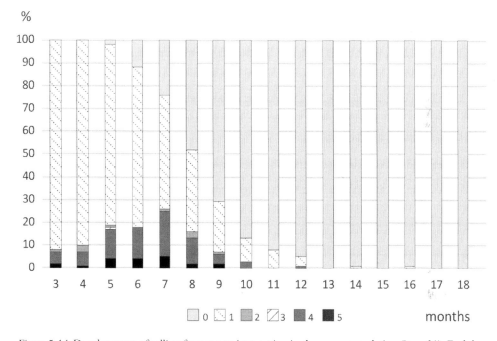

Figure 5.14 Development of rolling from prone into supine in the norm population (item 31). Each bar represents 100 infants. The numbers in the legends denote the scores of the item.

Figure 5.14 shows the development of rolling from prone into supine in the norm population. At three to four months, 7% of infants are able to roll from prone into supine; at five to seven months, 17% to 25% of infants are able to perform this action, unilaterally or bilaterally. Thereafter, the proportion of infants who have alternative ways to move around in space gradually increases, making rolling from prone into supine a non-preferred movement strategy.

32. *Variation in crawling (V)*

The repertoire of crawling movements (i.e., movements used during abdominal crawling or crawling on hands and knees) (item 29: scores 3 and 4) is assessed.

The size of the repertoire of movements of both sides of the body is taken into account (Video 5.10). This implies that the presence of a typical movement repertoire on one side of the body in combination with a limited repertoire on the other side results in the classification 'insufficient variation'.

0 = does not show progression while prone (item 29: score 1 or 2)

1 = insufficient variation
2 = sufficient variation

Score 0   The infant does not show progression while prone. This means that the infant lies immobile, shows pre-crawling movements without body displacement or shows pivoting movements; the infant received score 1 or 2 at item 29. Note that score 0 does not imply a worse score than score 1 or 2; it simply denotes that the score is not taken into account in the calculation of IMP scores.

Score 1   The infant shows only a limited repertoire of crawling movements in a limited number of movement combinations in neck, trunk, arms, and/or legs. One example is crawling movements in which the pelvic girdle moves *en bloc* in combination with lateroflexion of the trunk.

Score 2   The infant shows crawling with various combinations of movements in neck, trunk, arms, and/or legs.

33.   *Adaptability of crawling (A)*

Adaptability of crawling refers to the infant's ability to select the most appropriate and efficient crawling movements in each situation (see Video 5.11).

If an infant uses multiple ways of crawling (e.g., belly crawling and crawling on hands and knees), scoring is based on the overall ability to select the most efficient pattern.

0 = does not show progression while prone (item 29: score 1 or 2)

Majority of movements:

1 = no selection
2 = adaptive selection

Score 0   The infant does not show progression while prone. This means that the infant lies immobile, shows pre-crawling movements without body displacement or shows pivoting movements; the infant received score 1 or 2 at item 29. Note that score 0 does not imply a worse score than score 1 or 2; it simply denotes that the score is not taken into account in the calculation of IMP scores.

Score 1   During the majority of crawling sequences, the infant does not select specific and efficient movement strategies out of the crawling repertoire. In general, the infant explores various crawling strategies. Score 1 is also assigned if the infant has a motor repertoire that consists of only one stereotyped motor pattern.

Score 2   During the majority of crawling sequences, the infant selects specific and efficient crawling strategies out of the repertoire available; the strategies suit the specific situations. A prerequisite for adaptive selection is that the repertoire consists of more than one motor strategy.

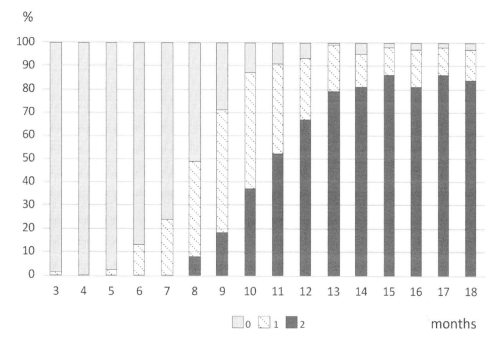

Figure 5.15 Development of adaptability of crawling in the norm population (item 33). Each bar represents 100 infants. The numbers in the legends denote the scores of the item.

Figure 5.15 shows the development of adaptability of crawling in the norm population. The ability to crawl, with the belly on or off the support surface, emerges at five months, but adaptive crawling emerges first at eight months. At that age, 8% of infants show adaptive crawling. The proportion of infants showing adaptive crawling gradually increases with increasing age. At 14 months, its prevalence stabilizes at 81% to 86%. This suggests that 15% to 20% of infants do not develop adaptive crawling movements, at least not up until the age of 18 months.

6 Assessment of motor behaviour in the sitting position

This chapter contains the description of the IMP items assessed in the sitting position. Sitting on the floor or on a mattress on the floor is evaluated in all infants; assessment in this position cannot be skipped. In young infants, sitting implies supported sitting; in older infants, independent sitting is evaluated. Putting infants who cannot sit independently into a supported sitting position has no negative impact on the infant's development. Rather, evidence indicates that putting infants who cannot sit independently in a supported sitting position to challenge their postural skills is associated with a favourable effect on motor development (Hadders-Algra et al. 1997, Dirks et al. 2016).

Procedure

The infant's spontaneous motor behaviour while sitting is assessed for several minutes, depending on the age and the functional abilities of the infant (Video 6.1). As mentioned earlier, sitting is assessed on the floor or on a mattress on the floor. It is not assessed on a chair, stool, bench, or the caregiver's lap. Young infants or infants with neurological impairment who cannot sit up independently are placed in a sitting position via the pull-to-sit manoeuvre: the infant lying in a supine position is pulled into sit by gentle traction on both wrists. If the infant has poor head balancing capacities, the examiner performs the pulling manoeuvre with one hand, leaving her other hand free to guide the infant's head movements. If the infant exhibits hyperextension of neck, trunk, or hips during pull-to-sit, the examiner also carries the pulling manoeuvre out with one hand, leaving her other hand free to apply some pressure on the infant's pubic region.

For an infant who is not able to sit independently, motor behaviour of the head is assessed first. The assessor supports the infant's trunk by placing her hands just below the infant's armpits and pays attention to the infant's head movements. Head support is only provided when head control is severely limited. When the infant does not show spontaneous head movements in all directions, the assessor elicits head movements by presentation of her face or an attractive toy.

Next, sitting behaviour is tested. If the infant requires little external support to remain in a sitting position, the infant's ability to sit independently is assessed: the examiner gently removes her supporting hands from the infant and observes subsequent behaviour. If the infant topples over, the examiner prevents falling by catching him. The infant is repositioned in a proper sitting position, and the procedure of the removal of the supporting hands is repeated several times. To orient the infant's attention forward, it may be helpful to put an interesting object on the floor in front of him or to let him hold an object in his hand. This assists in the assessment of sitting, particularly in infants with a tendency to hyperextend neck and trunk.

If the infant is able to sit independently, the standard sitting position consists of sitting on the buttocks in so-called 'long-leg sitting', with or without some abduction of the legs. Sitting behaviour is evaluated by the presentation of toys at various locations. First, toys are presented in front of the infant at close distance. If the infant is able to grasp these toys, toys are presented a little farther away. They are presented within reach at various distances and in various directions – i.e., semi-forward, lateral, and semi-backward on both sides of the body and at various heights (on the support surface, shoulder height, above shoulder height). Toy presentation at various locations aims at the evaluation of the size of the repertoire of sitting postures and movements, including trunk rotation (variation) and the ability to adapt sitting to the specifics of the situation (adaptability). To elicit trunk rotation, interesting objects are placed halfway behind the infant, on the floor or a bit higher (maximum height is nipple line), or the caregiver is asked to attract the infant's attention.

Sitting behaviour of infants who are able to sit and sit up independently is observed during spontaneous motor activity while they are moving into various body positions, such as crawling and sitting. If the infant only adopts W sitting (i.e., sits between the knees with the legs in a W form, which may credit for item 43 'getting into sitting position'), the infant also needs be put into sitting on his buttocks. This position is obligatory for items 36 ('sitting ability') and 37 ('posture of trunk while sitting independently').

For infants who can sit independently, sitting on the floor or mattress is also a good position to evaluate reaching, grasping, and manipulation in a sitting position as an add-on to (not as a substitute for!) sitting on the caregiver's lap (items 66–74).

34.   *Control of head movements (P)*

Control of head movements in a sitting position refers to the ability of the infant to master the movements of his head in this position. Basically, two types of head movements can be distinguished: (1) balancing head movements: that is, movements that aim at keeping the head upright (these movements are generally small in amplitude) and (2) goal-directed movements of the head: that is, movements to turn the head in various directions.

The control of head movements is assessed in supported sitting in infants who cannot sit independently; in infants who have mastered the skill of independent sitting, the control of head movements is assessed in sitting without support. When the infant shows no or few spontaneous movements of his head, and it is still unclear to what extent he is able to control his head movements, specific head movements are elicited. The infant's abilities may be unclear: for example, when his head is preferentially turned to one side. Head movements may be elicited by presenting the examiner's face or attractive toys to the infant in different head-turning positions (Video 6.1).

> 1 = cannot control head movements
> 2 = can control head movements to a limited extent
> 3 = can control head movements

Score 1   The infant does not lift his head against gravity in a sitting position. This means that the head either hangs limply down (to one side, forwards, or backwards) or is pulled back in stereotyped hyperextension (Figure 6.1A).

Score 2   The infant shows some capacity to lift and turn his head and to maintain it in a limited number of positions, but he is not fully able to turn his head in all directions and cannot maintain it in any desired position. The limited capacity to control head movements usually is accompanied by wobbling movements of the head (Video 6.1).

Score 3   The infant keeps his head upright, turns his head in any desired direction, and maintains it in any desired position; an occasionally occurring small wobbly movement of the head may be present (Figure 6.1B, Video 6.1).

> Note: 'control of head movements' is based on the overall performance while sitting; this means that in this performance item, the general principle of the performance (P) domain, 'score the best performance observed', is not applied.

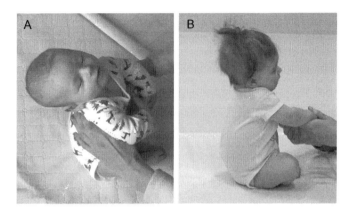

Figure 6.1 Control of head movements (item 34). (A) Infant of three months, who cannot control head movements; (B) infant of five months, who can control head movements.

Figure 6.2 shows the development of the control of head movements in a sitting position in the norm population. At three months, the majority of infants (86%) can control their head movements to a limited extent, whereas 3% of infants cannot control

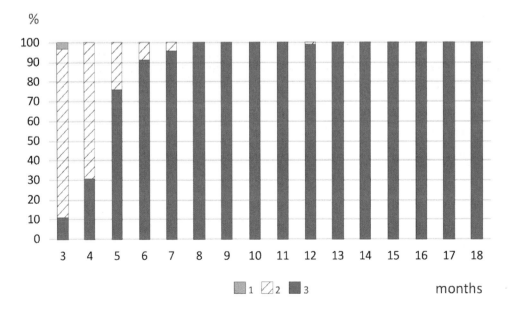

Figure 6.2 Development of control of head movements while sitting in the norm population (item 34). Each bar represents 100 infants. The numbers in the legends denote the scores of the item.

their head movements, and 11% have full control of head movements. The full control of head movements rapidly increases with increasing age: 31% of four-months-olds, 76% of five-months-olds, and 91% of six-months-olds are able to control their head movements.

35. *Position of head while sitting: presence of prevailing head position to one side (S)*

The presence of an asymmetry in prevailing head position is assessed (Video 6.2).

   1 = strongly prevailing head position to the R/L
   2 = moderately prevailing head position to the R/L
   3 = no or mildly prevailing head position to one side

Score 1   The infant keeps his head turned to one side virtually all time. The presentation of an interesting face or toy does not elicit head-turning movements across the midline to the contralateral side: R=right and L=left.
Score 2   The infant keeps his head turned substantially longer to one side than to the other side. Score 2 implies that notwithstanding the dominance of the head being turned into one direction, turning of the head across the midline may be elicited by presenting an interesting face or toy in that direction: R=right and L=left.
Score 3   The head is equally or almost equally often turned to the right and to the left side or is kept in the midline.

   Figure 6.3 shows that at three months, 28% of the infants have a preferred head position to one side, including 7% having a strongly prevailing head position. With increasing

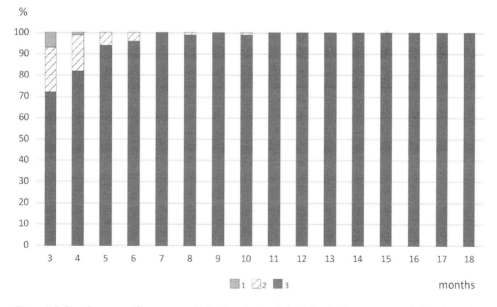

Figure 6.3 Development of asymmetry in head position while sitting in the norm population (item 35). Each bar represents 100 infants. The numbers in the legends denote the scores of the item.

age, the prevalence of asymmetric head position while sitting rapidly decreases to 4% at six months and 0% at seven months.

36.   *Sitting ability (P)*

Infants who are able to sit independently are placed in sitting position (on their buttocks) or may spontaneously adopt sitting positions. Infants who are not able to sit independently are put into a sitting position and provided with enough postural support that the infant is able to show his postural capacities. (See the procedures section in the chapter's introduction; Video 6.3.) Infants who spontaneously only sit between the knees with their legs in W form are put on their buttocks.

    1 = cannot sit independently
    2 = sits with extreme pelvis anteflexion (belly touching upper legs), with arms in propped position; cannot sit upright
    3 = sits independently for at least five seconds; cannot shift weight
    4 = sits independently, is able to shift weight, but shows no or minor trunk rotation
    5 = sits independently, is able to shift weight and to rotate the trunk

Score 1   The infant is not able to sit independently.

Score 2   The infant has minimal capacity to sit without help. He can only sit with extreme pelvis anteflexion with his belly touching his upper legs and his arms in propped position (Figure 6.4A). The infant is placed in this position by the examiner. To pass the item, the infant needs to maintain this position for at least five seconds. The infant is not able to sit upright or without arm support.

Score 3   The infant sits independently and more or less upright for at least five seconds before he loses balance; the infant cannot be left alone while sitting on his buttocks. Independent sitting implies being able to sit with or without support of arms and hands. A score 3 is also given to an infant who is able to sit independently for more than five seconds but is unable to shift weight without losing balance.

Score 4   The infant sits independently on his buttocks and is able to shift weight but shows no trunk rotation or trunk rotation of less than 40 degrees (Figure 6.4B). The infant may be left alone while sitting on his buttocks.

Score 5   The infant sits independently on his buttocks and is able to shift weight and to rotate the trunk least 40 degrees while reaching for toys in various directions, at various distances, and at various heights (Figure 6.4C). The observation of clear trunk rotation to one side is sufficient to achieve score 5. Trunk rotation is only credited when performed without arm support.

    Note: infants who lack the capacity to rotate their trunks while sitting are often able to rotate towards toys by using pelvic and/or leg movements. To achieve score 5, rotations must be present in the trunk.

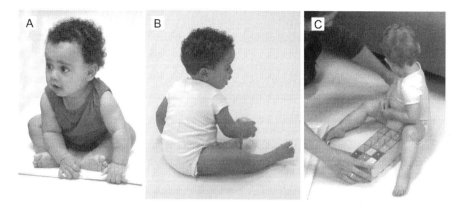

Figure 6.4 Sitting ability (item 36). (A) Six-month-old boy sits with extreme pelvis anteflextion with arms in propped position; (B) 12-month-old boy sits independently but shows limited trunk rotation; (C) 12-month-old girl sits independently and is able to rotate the trunk ≥40 degrees.

Figure 6.5 shows the development of sitting ability in the norm population. Some exceptional infants manage to sit for more than five seconds independently before the age of six months. At six months, 25% of infants have achieved this skill, including 6% who also can shift weight while sitting. The ability to sit independently with weight shifting – with or without rotation – gradually increases: 12% of seven-month-olds, 42% of eight-month-olds, 82% of nine-month-olds, and more than 90% of infants aged at least ten months have achieved this skill. Trunk rotation of at least 40 degrees emerges at eight months; from ten months onwards, it is shown by 30% to 50% of the infants.

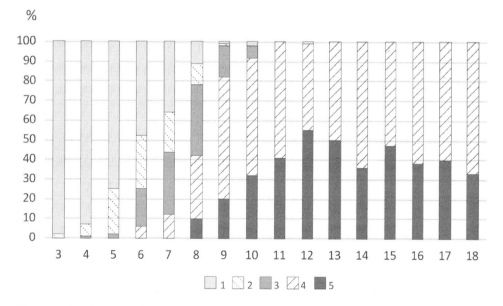

Figure 6.5 Development of sitting ability in the norm population (item 36). Each bar represents 100 infants. The numbers in the legends denote the scores of the item.

37.   *Posture of trunk while sitting independently (P)*

Sitting behaviour during independent sitting is observed. The best sitting posture during the assessment is recorded. The best sitting posture is not necessarily the most frequently occurring sitting posture.

This item can only be assessed if the infant shows some form of independent sitting: that is, if he achieved at least score 3 at item 36. For a proper assessment of trunk posture while sitting, the infant needs to sit on his buttocks in the so-called long-legs position.

   0 = cannot sit independently (item 36: score 1 or 2)

   1 = round back
   2 = straight back

Score 0   The infant is not able to sit independently; the infant received score 1 or 2 at item 36. Note that score 0 does not imply a worse score than score 1 or 2; it simply denotes that the score is not taken into account in the calculation of IMP scores.

Score 1   The infant sits with a rounded back (Figure 6.6A, B). This means a collapsed, floppy posture or 'sacral' sitting: that is, sitting with reclined pelvis and flexed trunk (van der Heide et al. 2005). Infants who show 'sacral' sitting during long-leg sitting tend to compensate for the 'sacral' posture with knee flexion. This means that attention should be paid to knee flexion as this may mask 'sacral' sitting. Infants who spontaneously sit only between the knees with the legs in W form always receive score 1.
Score 2   The infant sits with a straight back with or without evident lumbar lordosis (Figure 6.6C).

Figure 6.7 shows the development of trunk posture while sitting independently in the norm population. At the age of six months, 25% of infants can sit independently for at least five seconds; 44% of these infants sit with a straight trunk. The ability to sit

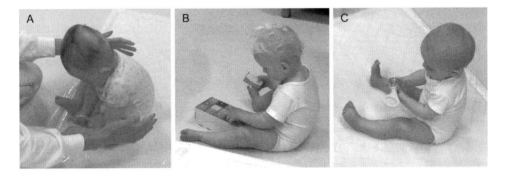

Figure 6.6 Posture of trunk during independent sitting (item 37). (A) Infant of eight months with round back; (B) infant of 14 months with round back; (C) infant of nine months with straight back.

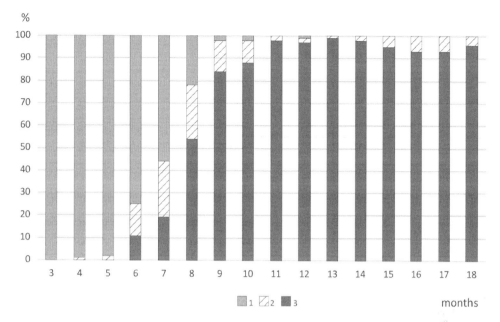

Figure 6.7 Development of trunk posture during independent sitting in the norm population (item 37). Each bar represents 100 infants. The numbers in the legends denote the scores of the item.

with a straight trunk gradually increases with increasing age: at eight months, about half the infants sit with a straight trunk; at nine months, 84% of the infants do; and from 11 months onwards, more than 90% of the infants do.

38. *Posture of trunk and legs while sitting: presence of asymmetry (S)*

The presence of an asymmetry in trunk and leg postures while sitting on the buttocks unsupported is assessed (Video 6.4). For infants who cannot sit without help, the presence of the supporting hands of the examiner interferes with the assessment of trunk asymmetry, thereby precluding the assessment of this item.

0 = cannot sit independently (item 36: score 1 or 2)

1 = strong asymmetry, R/L worst side
2 = moderate asymmetry, R/L worst side
3 = no or mild asymmetry

Score 0   The infant is not able to sit independently; the infant received score 1 or 2 at item 36. Note that score 0 does not imply a worse score than score 1 or 2; it simply denotes that the score is not taken into account in the calculation of IMP scores.

Score 1   The infant shows a strong asymmetry in trunk and or leg postures while sitting. For example, the infant collapses consistently to one side, or one leg shows consistently clear stereotyped behaviour, including, for instance, ankle plantarflexion and clawing or stereotyped dorsiflexion of the first toe. The worst side is the side with the stereotyped leg postures or the side to which the infant collapses: R=right and L=left.

Score 2   The infant shows a moderate asymmetry in trunk and leg postures while sitting. The infant shows the postures described at score 1 but also shows some other postures. The worst side is the side with stereotyped leg postures or the side to which the infant collapses: R=right and L=left.

Score 3   No or minimal asymmetries in trunk and leg postures are present while sitting.

39.   *Posture and movements of upper extremities during sitting or supported sitting: presence of asymmetry (S)*

The presence of asymmetry in posture and movements of the upper extremities during supported or unsupported sitting is assessed (Video 6.5). The infant may sit on his buttocks, or he may sit between his knees with his legs in W form. This item is not assessed in infants who can only sit independently to a limited extent (see score 0).

   0 = the infant can sit independently to a limited extent (item 36: score 2 or 3)

   1 = strong asymmetry, R/L worst side
   2 = moderate asymmetry, R/L worst side
   3 = no or mild asymmetry

Score 0   The infant can sit independently to a limited extent, implying that the infant sits with extreme pelvis flexion with arms propped (item 36: score 2) or is able to sit independently but cannot shift weight (item 36: score 3). Score 0 is not taken into account in the calculation of IMP scores. Note: score 0 is not assigned when item 36 achieved score 1.

Score 1   The infant shows a strong asymmetry in upper extremity posture and movements while sitting. For example, the infant shows a stereotyped flexion of the elbow with or without fisting of the hand or a consistent difference in involvement of arms in manual play activity and postural support, and the infant does not or only exceptionally shows other arm postures. In strong asymmetries, the worst functioning arm is participating less in both manual and supportive activities: R=right and L=left.

Score 2   The infant shows a moderate asymmetry in upper extremity posture and movements while sitting. For example, the infant shows frequent fisting of one hand or a marked difference in involvement of arms in postural support and also shows other arm postures. Infants with a moderate asymmetry in arm activity often use the worst side for postural support, while the contralateral part is used for manual activities. This, however, is not a law of the Medes and Persians: R=right and L=left.

Score 3   The infant shows no or a mild asymmetry in posture and movements of the arms and hands while sitting: for example, the infant may show occasionally fisting of one hand or a minor difference in involvement of the arms in postural support.

40.   *Uses arms for voluntary activities (P)*

This item addresses the degree to which the infant is able to use his arms for voluntary activities while sitting independently. The item can only be assessed if the infant shows some form of independent sitting: that is, if he has at least score 3 at item 36.

0 = cannot sit independently (item 36: score 1 or 2)

1 = uses one or two arms for postural support, does not use arms for voluntary activity
2 = uses one arm for postural support, uses other arm for voluntary activity
3 = uses both arms for voluntary activity, does not need arms for postural support

Score 0   The infant is not able to sit independently; the infant scored 1 or 2 at item 36. Note that score 0 does not imply a worse score than score 1 or 2; it simply denotes that the score is not taken into account in the calculation of IMP scores.

Score 1   The infant is able to sit independently for at least five seconds (item 36: score 3) and uses one or two arms for postural support. The arm or arms are not used for voluntary activity such as playing with toys.

Score 2   The infant uses one arm for postural support while sitting and uses the other arm and hand for voluntary activity, such as playing with toys.

Score 3   The infant uses both arms arbitrarily for voluntary activity, such as playing with toys, and does not need arms and hands for postural support while sitting.

Figure 6.8 shows the development of voluntary arm use while sitting independently in the norm population. Voluntary use of one or two arms while sitting independently emerges at six months. The ability rapidly increases with increasing age: it is present in 13% of six-month-olds, 35% of seven-month-olds, 62% of eight-month-olds, and more than 95% of infants of at least nine months.

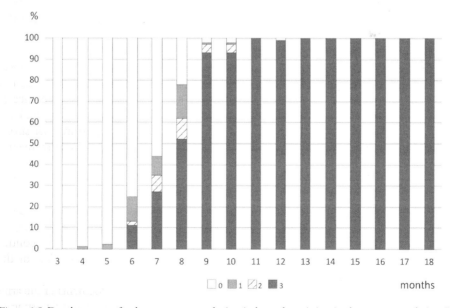

Figure 6.8 Development of voluntary arm use during independent sitting in the norm population (item 40). Each bar represents 100 infants. The numbers in the legends denote the scores of the item.

41.   Variation in sitting movements (V)

The size of the repertoire of sitting movements is assessed (Video 6.7). Sitting movements imply the small movements of neck, trunk, legs, and arms used to vary and adjust sitting position. The item can only be assessed if the infant shows some form of independent sitting: that is, if he has at least score 3 at item 36.

0 = cannot sit independently (item 36: score 1 or 2)

1 = insufficient variation
2 = sufficient variation

Score 0   The infant is not able to sit independently; the infant scored 1 or 2 at item 36. Note that score 0 does not imply a worse score than score 1 or 2; it simply denotes that the score is not taken into account in the calculation of IMP scores.

Score 1   The infant shows a limited repertoire of movements of neck, trunk, and legs while sitting in a limited number of combinations (Figure 6.9). For example, the infant sits virtually consistently with a stiff, straight trunk, or the infant sits most of the time in a collapsed position, or one or both legs show a stereotyped postures. Infants who spontaneously only use the W position to sit and those who move immediately into W position when the examiners put them on their buttocks, also are assigned score 1. The presence of repetitive, stereotyped, circular wrist and ankle movements or flapping arm movements while sitting is also regarded as an expression of insufficient variation.

Score 2   The infant shows a sufficiently large repertoire of small movements of neck, trunk, and legs in various combinations while sitting (Figure 6.10).

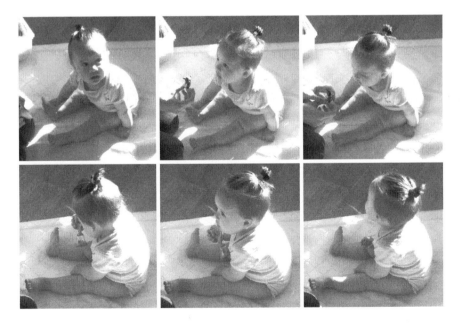

Figure 6.9 Insufficient variation in sitting movements in an infant of seven months (item 41)

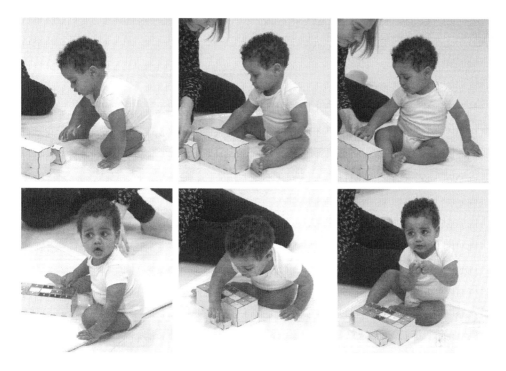

Figure 6.10 Sufficient variation in sitting movements in an infant of 12 months (item 41)

42.   *Adaptability of sitting movements (A)*

Adaptability of sitting movements refers to the infant's ability to select the most appropriate and efficient sitting postures and movements in each situation (Video 6.7). The infant's repertoire may include variants of sitting on the buttocks and/or variants of W-position sitting.

The item can only be assessed if the infant shows some form of independent sitting: that is, if he has at least score 3 at item 36.

   0 = cannot sit independently (item 36: score 1 or 2)

Majority of movements:

   1 = no adaptive selection
   2 = adaptive selection

Score 0   The infant is not able to sit independently; the infant received score 1 or 2 at item 36. Note that score 0 does not imply a worse score than score 1 or 2; it simply denotes that the score is not taken into account in the calculation of IMP scores.

Score 1   During the majority of sitting movements, the infant does not select specific and efficient strategies out of the sitting repertoire adjusted to the situation. In general, the infant explores various adjustment strategies with some trials leading to error. The latter may result in loosing sitting balance. Score 1 is also assigned if the infant has a motor repertoire that consists of only one strategy and if the infant is only able to sit more or less upright for a few seconds (item 36: score 3).

Score 2   During the majority of sitting movements, the infant selects specific and efficient postural adjustments out of the repertoire of postural adjustments. This results in sitting behaviour that is predominantly integrated into the infant's play behaviour while sitting. A prerequisite for adaptive selection is that the repertoire consists of more than one motor strategy.

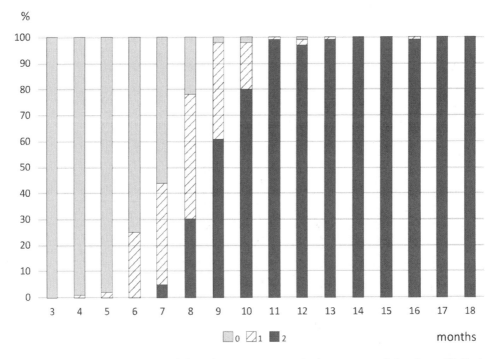

Figure 6.11 Development of adaptability of sitting movements in the norm population (item 42). Each bar represents 100 infants. The numbers in the legends denote the scores of the item.

Figure 6.11 shows the development of adaptability of sitting movements in the norm population. Adaptability of sitting movements emerges at seven months: a minority of the infants who are able to sit independently are able use adaptive sitting movements. After seven months, the proportion of infants showing adaptive sitting movements rapidly increases: 30% of eight-month-olds show adaptive sitting movements, as do 61% of nine-month-olds and 80% of ten-month-olds. Finally, 97% to 100% of infants aged at least 11 months use adaptive sitting movements.

43.   *Getting into sitting position (P)*

Getting into sitting position is the action of bringing oneself from supine or prone position into a sitting position on the floor or on a mattress on the floor (Figure 6.12A). It may also consist of the action of getting oneself seated on the floor or on a mattress on the floor from a standing position (Figure 6.12B). Younger infants only employ a sitting-up strategy to get seated; older infants may use both sitting up and sitting down to get seated on the floor. Both sitting on the buttocks and sitting on the heels or between the knees with the legs in W form are considered sitting positions here (Figure 6.12C, D). 'Half sitting' (Figure 6.13) is not regarded as a sitting position.

  1 = does not sit up or sit down independently
  2 = does sit up or sit down independently

Score 1   The infant does not sit up from a supine or prone position without the help of the examiner. The infant also does not sit down independently from a standing position.
Score 2   The infant sits up independently from a supine or prone position or sits down independently from a standing position.

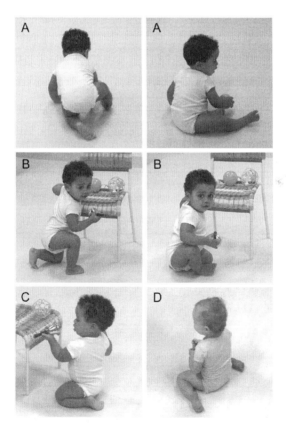

Figure 6.12 Various ways to get into a sitting position (item 43). (A) From prone (crawling) to sitting; (B) from standing to sitting; (C) sitting on the heels; (D) sitting between the heels in a W-position.

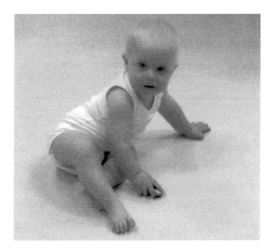

Figure 6.13 Infant of eight months in a half-sitting position; this performance does not credit for score 2 at item 43.

Figure 6.14 shows the development of getting into a sitting position in the norm population. At six to seven months, some exceptional infants are able to get into a sitting position, and at eight months, 14% have achieved this skill. After the age of eight months, the ability to get into a sitting position rapidly increases with increasing age: at ten months, 60% get into sitting position, at 11 to 12 months, 84% to 87% do, and in infants aged at least 13 months, this proportion rises to 98% or more.

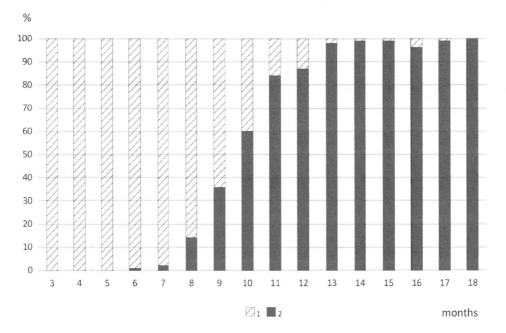

Figure 6.14 Development of getting into a sitting position in the norm population (item 43). Each bar represents 100 infants. The numbers in the legends denote the scores of the item.

44.   *Variation in getting into a sitting position (V)*

The size of the repertoire of sitting up and sitting down movements is assessed (Video 6.8). Both sitting on the buttocks and sitting on the heels or between the knees with the legs in W form are considered sitting positions. Variation of getting into a sitting position can only be assessed when the infant has performed the action more than once.

> 0 = the infant did not show or only once showed sitting up or sitting down movements

> 1 = insufficient variation
> 2 = sufficient variation

Score 0   The infant does not show sitting up or sitting down movements or shows these activities only once, which precludes the assessment of variation in this behaviour. Note that score 0 does not imply a worse score than score 1 or 2; it simply denotes that the score is not taken into account in the calculation of IMP scores.

Score 1   The infant shows a limited repertoire of sitting up or sitting down strategies, during which legs, arms, and trunk are used in a limited number of movement combinations with little variation in movement sequencing. Examples are sitting up movements in which the pelvic region of the body and the upper legs are moved *en bloc* and consistent asymmetries.

Score 2   The infant shows sitting up or sitting down strategies with various combinations of movements in legs, arms, and trunk. In addition, the movements are characterized by variation in movement sequence.

45.   *Adaptability of getting into a sitting position (A)*

Adaptability of sitting up and sitting down behaviour refers to the infant's ability to select the most appropriate and efficient movements to sit up or to sit down in each situation (Video 6.9). Adaptability of getting into a sitting position can only be assessed when the infant has performed the action more than once. Both sitting on the buttocks and sitting on the heels or between the knees with the legs in W form are considered sitting positions (Figure 6.12).

> 0 = the infant did not show or only once showed sitting up or sitting down movements

Majority of movements:

> 1 = no adaptive selection
> 2 = adaptive selection

Score 0   The infant does not show sitting up or sitting down movements or shows these activities only once, which precludes the assessment of the variation in this behaviour. Note that score 0 does not imply a worse score than score 1

or 2; it simply denotes that the score is not taken into account in the calculation of IMP scores.

Score 1   During the majority of movements, the infant does not select specific and
efficient strategies out of the repertoire of getting into sitting movements. In
general, the infant explores various strategies to sit up or sit down. Score 1
is also assigned if the infant has a motor repertoire that consists of only one
strategy.

Score 2   During the majority of movements, the infant selects specific and efficient
strategies to sit up or sit down out of the repertoire of getting into sitting
movements. If the infant shows adaptive and efficient movements when sitting
up but not when sitting down (e.g., the infant 'crashes down' from standing),
the infant is assigned score 2. This means that performance during sitting up
contributes more to adaptability of getting into sitting position than sitting
down. A prerequisite for adaptive selection is that the repertoire consists of
more than one motor strategy.

Figure 6.15 shows the development of adaptability of getting into a sitting position
in the norm population. Adaptability of getting into a sitting position emerges at eight
months, when 8% of infants have achieved this ability. Thereafter, the proportion of
infants showing adaptive movements while getting into a sitting position increases with
increasing age. At ten months, 41% of infants move adaptively into sitting position, and
at 12 months, 80% have achieved this ability. The proportion of infants aged 13 to 18
months moving adaptively into sitting position stabilizes at 87% to 94%.

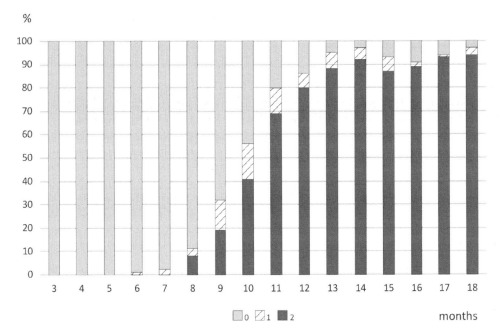

Figure 6.15 Development of adaptability of getting into a sitting position in the norm population (item
45). Each bar represents 100 infants. The numbers in the legends denote the scores of the item.

46. Bottom shuffling (V)

Bottom shuffling is a sliding action with the trunk erect and the hips flexed, the weight being taken on the buttocks or on one buttock and a flexed lower limb; the feet or hands or both may be used for propulsion (Peiper 1963, Robson 1970). This specific way of locomotion may be part of typical development, but stereotyped bottom shuffling is associated with an increased risk of developmental motor disorders such as CP (Robson 1970, Largo et al. 1985, Bottos et al. 1989).

The item can only be assessed if the infant shows some form of independent sitting: i.e., if he has at least score 4 at item 36.

0 = cannot sit independently (item 36: score 1, 2, or 3)

1 = bottom shuffling, apart from walking, is the only strategy to move around
2 = no bottom shuffling present or bottom shuffling present as one of the strategies to move around

Score 0 The infant is not able to sit independently or only sits independently for a few seconds; the infant received score 1 to 3 at item 36. Note that score 0 does not imply a worse score than score 1 or 2; it simply denotes that the score is not taken into account in the calculation of IMP scores.

Score 1 The infant shows either bottom shuffling or walking to move around. The infant does not show abdominal crawling or crawling on all fours (Figure 6.16, Video 6.10).

Score 2 The infant does not show bottom shuffling or bottom shuffling is one of the strategies which the infant uses to move around: that is, the infant also uses other strategies to move around, such as abdominal crawling, crawling, or walking.

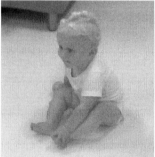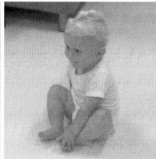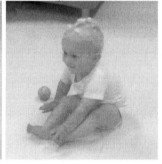

Figure 6.16 The infant moves forward by means of bottom shuffling (item 46)

7 Assessment of motor behaviour while standing and walking

This chapter describes the IMP items assessed while standing and walking. Standing and walking are only assessed in infants aged at least six months. In infants younger than six months, the calculator of the IMP app automatically assigns the scores associated with not being able to stand or walk.

Procedure

The infant's spontaneous motor behaviour while standing and walking is assessed for several minutes, depending on the age, the functional abilities, and the mood of the infant (Video 7.1). Infants who have mastered the ability to walk without help are usually eager to walk around, pick up toys and bring them to their caregiver, and play with a ball. To facilitate the evaluation of walking, including adaptability and balancing capacities while walking, the presence of a thin examination mattress on the floor is recommended. In addition, we suggest not tidying up the 'messy' situation with toys scattered around the room that spontaneously develops during the assessment – tidying up is performed after completion of the assessment. The 'messy' floor situation assists in the evaluation of the infant's capacities to adapt walking movements to the environment.

Infants who are close to the ability to stand are encouraged to stand up. This may be achieved by putting attractive toys on a table, stool, couch, or chair, the surface of which should be at the height of the infant's waist. The examiner encourages the infant to stand up and get hold of the toys, but she does not manually assist the infant in getting up. The encouragement works best if the examiner plays with the toys and invites the infant to join in the play. If the infant is successful in standing up, the infant is allowed to play a while with the objects. Next, the examiner puts the objects on the floor and encourages the infant to move down and retrieve the toys. When the infant has returned to a sitting or prone position, she puts the toy on the chair again, challenging the infant to stand up again. This sequence of standing up and getting down is repeated multiple times, preferably at different spots (table, couch, chair), allowing for the assessment of variation and adaptability of standing up.

In infants aged six months or older who do not stand up, the ability to stand – that is, the ability to take weight on the legs – may be assessed by putting the infant in a standing position. The examiner may do this, but usually it is better to ask the caregiver to put the infant in a standing position as older infants generally are not fond of getting touched by strangers ('*noli me tangere*') (Hadders-Algra 2005). Weight bearing while standing is only credited when it is performed for at least five seconds.

If the infant is able to stand and walk independently, take care to elicit various ways of standing up: that is, take care that the child does not only stand up from a squatting position as the latter limits the ability to evaluate variation and adaptability in standing-up behaviour.

If the infant is able to stand independently, the ability to rotate the trunk is tested by presentation of toys in various directions (i.e., semi-forward, lateral, and semi-backward directions on both sides of the body) and at various heights (shoulder height, above shoulder height). Trunk rotation is only tested during unsupported standing, not while standing with support.

If an infant is able to bear weight on his legs but does not show independent walking, the infant's walking abilities are assessed by challenging him to walk while being held by the hand. First, the ability to walk while being held by two hands is tested. If that is successful, the ability to walk while held by only one hand is assessed. Again, it may be useful to ask for caregiver assistance in order to accomplish the assessment of 'walking with help'. Walking abilities may also be assessed with the help of a relatively low table or couch. The standing infant is challenged to hold on to the table or couch and to cruise towards attractive toys placed on the table or couch at some distance from the infant.

47.   Standing ability (P)

The infant's ability to stand is assessed (see procedures).

> 1 = cannot stand
> 2 = stands with help
> 3 = stands independently for a few seconds
> 4 = stands independently for more than ten seconds but rotates trunk to a minimal
> extent only
> 5 = stands independently and is able to rotate trunk

Score 1   The infant is not able to stand with or without support. Score 1 is automatically assigned to infants younger than six months.

Score 2   The infant stands with help (Figure 7.1A). Standing is achieved with support of a person or of furniture. The presence of standing behaviour implies that the legs bear weight. Standing while leaning with the hips flexed more than 60 degrees (i.e., with an almost horizontal trunk, leaning on the furniture or the caregiver) is not sufficient for score 2. Note that the way in which the infant performs the action (e.g., with firm or stiff legs) is not taken into account. To pass the item, the infant should be able to maintain the standing position for at least five seconds. The infant does not stand independently: that is, without external support.

Score 3   The infant stands independently (i.e., without external support) for a few seconds before losing balance. He maintains this position for more than two and fewer than ten seconds.

Score 4   The infant stands independently (i.e., without external support) for at least ten seconds and is able to shift weight but shows no or only minimal trunk rotation (Figure 7.1B, Video 7.2). Infants who are able to walk independently (item 51: score 4) with moderate to good balance (item 52: scores 2 and 3) also are assigned score 4, even when they do not stand still for at least ten seconds.

Score 5   The infant stands independently (i.e., without external support) and is able to shift weight and to rotate his trunk at least 30 degrees (Figure 7.1C, Video 7.2). Note that trunk rotation during standing with support is not sufficient for score 5; in order to be assigned score 5, trunk rotation should be performed during free stance.

Figure 7.2 shows the development of standing ability in the norm population. At six to seven months, about half the infants are able to stand with help, and at eight to

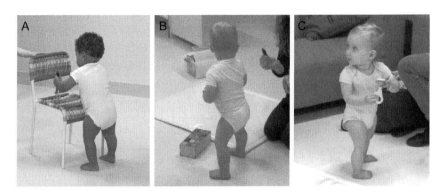

Figure 7.1 Standing ability (item 47). (A) Stands with help; (B) stands independently and rotates trunk to a minimal extent only; (C) stands independently and can rotate trunk at least 30 degrees.

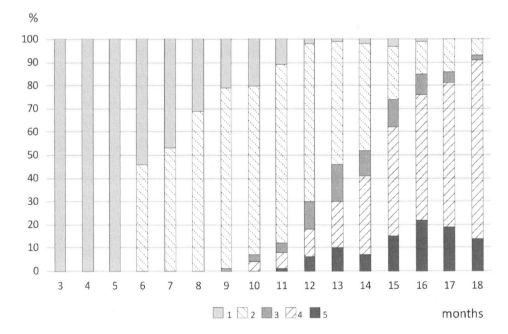

Figure 7.2 Development of standing ability in the norm population (item 47). Each bar represents 100 infants. The numbers in the legends denote the scores of the item.

nine months, about three-quarters of the infants have achieved this milestone. Standing independently slowly emerges at nine months, so that at 11 months, 12% of the infants are able to stand independently for at least a few seconds. The proportion of infants able to stand independently for at least ten seconds continues to increase steadily: 18% of 12-month-olds, 30% of 13-month-olds, 41% of 14-month-olds, 76% of 16-month-olds, and 91% of 18-month-olds have achieved this skill.

48. *Standing up (P)*

The infant's ability to stand up from the floor from a sitting or prone position may be assessed with the help of a small chair, stool, couch, or table (see procedures). Placing attractive toys on the chair, stool, couch, or table, encourages the infant to get to his knees and to stand up using the furniture (Video 7.3). An alternative way to elicit standing-up behaviour is to place attractive toys on the caregiver's lap. The caregiver encourages the infant to raise himself with the support of the caregiver's legs, but the caregiver is not allowed to assist the infant in his standing-up efforts (e.g., by pulling the infant up while holding his hands). Standing-up behaviour includes the movements preparatory to getting up, movements that especially may be observed in infants who cannot stand up independently without support of, for example, furniture.

If the infant is able to stand up independently without external support, standing up from sitting position on the floor may be elicited by presenting toys above the infant or by placing attractive objects on a chair, stool, or table situated at some distance from the infant. Note that rising up from squatting position is not regarded as standing up.

> 1 = cannot stand up
> 2 = gets on knees
> 3 = stands up independently with the use of, for example, furniture
> 4 = stands up independently without using furniture

Score 1   The infant does not stand up and does not get into a kneeling position. Score 1 is automatically assigned to infants younger than six months.

Score 2   The infant gets into a kneeling position while supporting himself with one or both hands (Touwen 1976). In the kneeling position, the buttocks do not touch the lower legs (Figure 7.3A, Video 7.3).

Score 3   The infant stands up independently, with the help of support surfaces, such as furniture or the caregiver; this means that the infant is able to achieve, with the help of a support surface, an erect standing position (Figure 7.3B, Video 7.3). External support (e.g., at the arms or buttocks by caregiver or assessor) is not allowed.

Score 4   The infant stands up independently without using support surfaces, such as furniture or caregiver (Figure 7.3C, Video 7.3). Note that the floor may be used as a support surface.

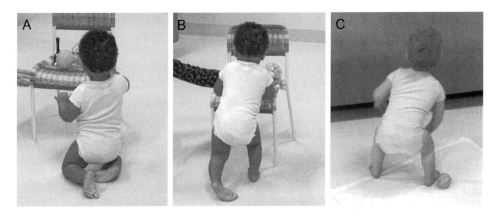

Figure 7.3 Standing up (item 48). (A) Gets on knees; (B) stands up independently with the use of furniture; (C) stands up independently without using furniture.

Figure 7.4 shows the development of standing up in the norm population.

At seven months, a few infants attempt to pull themselves into stance. At 8 to 11 months 5% to 13% of infants gets on their knees, whereas an increasing proportion of infants are able to pull themselves into standing position: 14% at eight months and 67% at 11 months. Standing up without the help of an external support surface emerges at 11 months. Thereafter, the proportion of infants able to stand up without help of external support gradually increases from 12% at 12 months to 84% at 18 months.

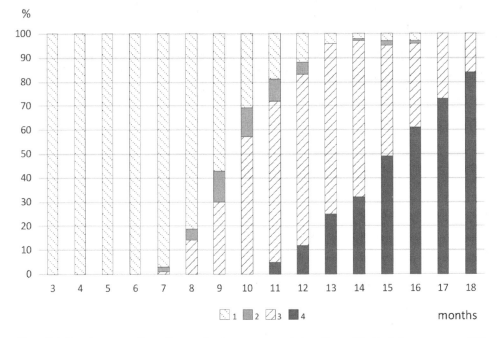

Figure 7.4 Development of standing up in the norm population (item 48). Each bar represents 100 infants. The numbers in the legends denote the scores of the item.

49. Variation in standing-up behaviour (V)

The size of the repertoire of movement strategies for standing up is assessed. Standing up may be performed with or without the help of a support surface (e.g., furniture, person). The focus of the assessment of variation is on the movements of the lower part of the body (hips, legs, and feet).

0 = the infant did not stand up or only stood up once

1 = insufficient variation
2 = sufficient variation

Score 0   The infant does not stand up or stands up only once, which precludes the assessment of variation in this behaviour. Note that score 0 does not imply a worse score than score 1 or 2; it simply denotes that the score is not taken into account in the calculation of IMP scores.

Score 1   The infant shows a limited repertoire of standing-up strategies, during which legs, arms, trunk, and head are used in a limited number of movement combinations (Video 7.4). Examples are stereotyped unilateral or bilateral leg extension movements, the latter of which are usually accompanied by strong pulling-up movements of the arms. Note that infants who just mastered the skill of standing up generally prefer one of the legs to initiate the standing-up action. This is not considered a stereotypy.

Score 2   The infant shows a sufficiently large repertoire of standing-up strategies, which consist of strategies during which various combinations of movements of legs, arms, trunk, and head are used (Figure 7.5, Video 7.4).

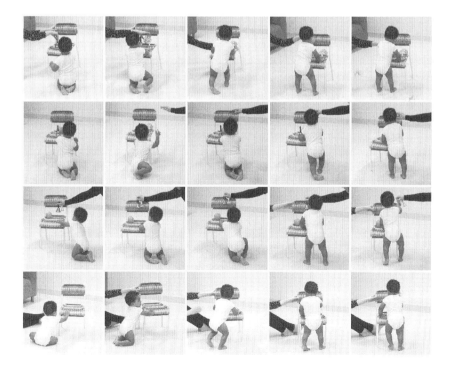

Figure 7.5 Infant of 12 months with sufficient variation in standing up movements (item 49)

50.   *Adaptability of standing-up behaviour (A)*

Adaptability of standing-up behaviour refers to the infant's ability to select efficient movements to stand up in each situation. The item can only be assessed if the infant shows some capacity to stand up independently: that is, if he has achieved at least score 3 at item 48. If an infant is able to stand up with help of, for example, furniture and to stand up independently, scoring is based on the overall ability to select the most efficient pattern. In general, this means that the infant mostly uses external support when standing up, implying that the assessment of adaptability is largely based on this activity.

0 = the infant did not stand up or only stood up once

Majority of movements:

1 = no adaptive selection
2 = adaptive selection

Score 0   The infant does not stand up or stands up only once, which precludes the assessment of variation in this behaviour. Note that score 0 does not imply a worse score than score 1 or 2; it simply denotes that the score is not taken into account in the calculation of IMP scores.

Score 1   During the majority of standing-up movements, the infant does not select specific and efficient strategies out of the repertoire of standing-up movements. In general, the infant explores various strategies to stand up (Video 7.5). Score 1 is also assigned if the infant has a motor repertoire that consists of only one strategy

Score 2   During the majority of standing-up movements, the infant selects specific and efficient strategies to stand up out of the repertoire of standing-up strategies (Video 7.5). A prerequisite for adaptive selection is that the repertoire consists of more than one motor strategy. The infant is also assigned score 2 if he shows adaptive standing-up behaviour when standing up with help (item 48: score 3) but shows non-adaptive standing up in the just-mastered activity of standing up without help (item 48: score 4).

Figure 7.6 shows the development of adaptability of standing-up movements in the norm population. Adaptability of standing-up movements emerges at eight or nine months. The proportion of infants using adaptive movements during standing up rapidly increases from 15% in ten-month-olds to 82% in 13-month-olds. Thereafter the prevalence of adaptive standing-up movements increases more slowly to more than 95% at 17 to 18 months.

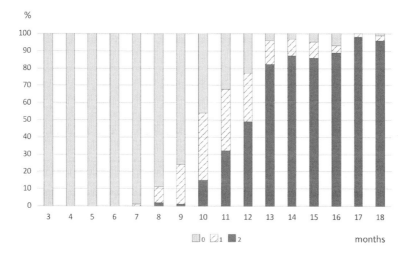

Figure 7.6 Development of adaptability of standing up in the norm population (item 50). Each bar represents 100 infants. The numbers in the legends denote the scores of the item.

51. *Walking (P)*

The infant's abilities to walk with or without help are assessed (see procedures; Video 7.6).

1 = cannot walk
2 = walks when receiving support by two hands
3 = walks when receiving support by one hand
4 = walks independently

Score 1   The infant is not able to walk with or without external support. Score 1 is automatically assigned to infants younger than six months.

Score 2   The infant is able to walk when receiving support from a person who holds both his hands. Provision of support of the infant's trunk or shoulders is not allowed. Score 2 is also assigned if the infant cruises along a piece of furniture which is held with both hands. For score 2, the infant needs to produce at least three steps.

Score 3   The infant is able to walk at least five steps when receiving support from a person who holds one of his hands, or the infant accomplishes a few steps independently. The infant does not walk independently for more than six steps without external support. Score 3 is also given if the infant cruises along a piece of furniture which is held with only one hand.

Score 4   The infant walks independently without external support for at least seven steps consecutively (Touwen 1976; Figure 7.7).

Figure 7.8 shows the development of walking in the norm population. The ability to walk supported by two hands emerges at seven months and walking independently at ten months. The proportion of infants able to walk without support steadily increases with increasing age, from 2% at ten months to 40% at 14 months, to 91% at 18 months.

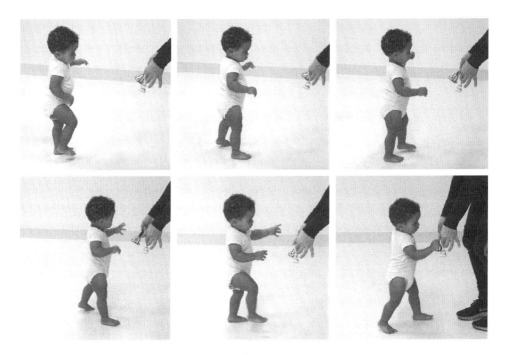

Figure 7.7 Infant of 12 months who just mastered independent walking (item 51)

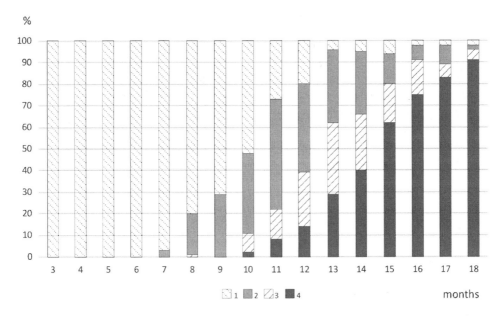

Figure 7.8 Development of walking in the norm population (item 51). Each bar represents 100 infants. The numbers in the legends denote the scores of the item.

52. *Balance while walking independently (P)*

The ability of the infant to maintain balance while walking independently is assessed (Video 7.7). Specific attention is paid to balancing capacities when the infant changes walking direction, stops walking and crosses the mattress, and tries to avoid objects on the floor. Limited balancing capacities may be reflected by the presence of correction movements of arms and trunk, swaying movements, walking with a broad base, and stumbling or falling (Hempel 1993).

0 = cannot walk independently (item 51: score 1, 2 or 3)

1 = poor balancing capacities
2 = moderate balancing capacities
3 = good balancing capacities

Score 0   The infant cannot walk independently; the infant received score 1, 2, or 3 at item 51. Note that score 0 does not imply a worse score than score 1 to 3; it simply denotes that the score is not taken into account in the calculation of IMP scores.

Score 1   The infant shows poor balancing capacities. The infant frequently loses balance, stumbles, and falls. The infant often shows swaying movements of trunk and arms in order to maintain balance. Score 1 is also assigned to infants who have just mastered the ability to walk seven steps independently but are unable to maintain balance for a longer period.

Score 2   The infant shows moderate balancing capacities. The infant shows swaying movements of trunk and arms and/or a broad walking base in order to maintain balance but does not fall or only falls once when stepping on the mattress or when faced with similar difficult balancing tasks. A broad walking base is reflected by placement of the feet laterally to the projection line of the pelvis onto the support surface.

Score 3   The infant shows good balancing capacities while walking independently. This is reflected by a medium-size walking base: that is, the feet are placed within the width of the pelvis. The infant may show some correction movements of arms and trunk in order to keep balance, in particular during complex motor activities. He does not stumble or fall.

Figure 7.9 shows the development of balance while walking in the norm population. In general, poor balance while walking reflects that the infant has little experience with walking; its prevalence is rather stable at 5% to 16% at 11 to 17 months. Only at ten months, when few infants are able to walk independently, and at 18 months, when the majority of infants have acquired some experience in walking independently, is the prevalence lower (2%). In the age period of 13 to 18 months, the large majority of infants who are able to walk independently have a moderate balancing capacity. Only a minor proportion of infants show good balancing capacities while walking from 13 to 18 months;

the prevalence of good balance during walking increases from 1% at 13 to 14 months to 29% at 18 months. The relatively late development of good balancing capacities while walking corresponds to the data on the onset of walking independently (Figure 7.8) and the notion that walking skills, including walking balance, are strongly dependent on walking experience (Ledebt and Bril 2000). The findings also indicate that it is relatively difficult for infants in the age range of the IMP to obtain score 3. However, the inclusion of 'difficult' items in a test is needed for the test's proper construction: that is, to avoid a so-called ceiling effect.

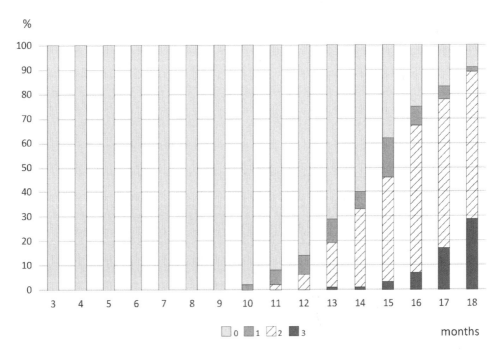

Figure 7.9 Development of balance during independent walking in the norm population (item 52). Each bar represents 100 infants. The numbers in the legends denote the scores of the item.

53. *Arm posture and movements while walking independently (P)*

Arm posture in novice walkers has been described as abducted and externally rotated at the shoulder and flexed at the elbow (Burnett and Johnson 1971). This posture is known as high-guard posture (Ledebt and Bril 2000). With increasing walking experience, shoulders are less abducted, and arms are lowered into semi-high guard. Finally, the infant does not need arm movements to maintain balance while walking and is able to use his arms for goal-directed movements (Hempel 1993). The item can only be assessed in infants who are able to walk independently: that is, who received score 4 at item 51.

0 = cannot walk independently (item 51: score 1, 2, or 3)

1 = high or semi-high guard

2 = arbitrary arm posture

Score 0   The infant cannot walk independently; the infant received score 1, 2, or 3 at item 51. Note that score 0 does not imply a worse score than score 1 or 2; it simply denotes that the score is not taken into account in the calculation of IMP scores.

Score 1   The infant shows consistently high- or semi-high-guard arm postures while walking independently and does not use his arms and hands for other activities (Figure 7.10, Videos 7.1 and 7.8). Carrying objects while holding the arms in high- or semi-high-guard position while walking is also assigned score 1.

Score 2   While walking independently, the infant shows arbitrary arm postures, which are incorporated into his play activities (Video 7.8). Often, this means that the infant is able to carry a toy below shoulder level while walking. The infant may only occasionally show high- or semi-high-guard arm postures.

Note: in case of asymmetrical performance, performance of the best side is recorded.

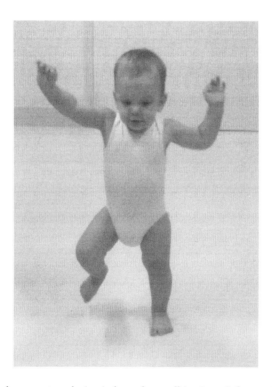

Figure 7.10 High guard arm posture during independent walking in an infant aged 13 months (item 53)

Figure 7.11 shows the development of arm posture and movements while walking independently in the norm population. The high- and semi-high-guard position is observed in 5% to 14% of infants aged 11 to 17 months, with the highest prevalence of

14% occurring at 14 months. At both 10 and 18 months, only a few infants show this arm posturing while walking independently. The prevalence of arbitrary arm postures and movements gradually increases with increasing age, from 2% at 11 months to 48% at 15 months to 90% at 18 months.

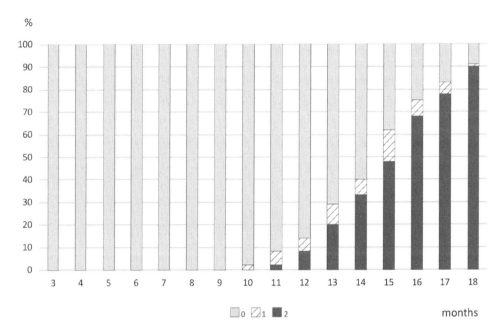

Figure 7.11 Development of arm posture and movements during independent walking in the norm population (item 53). Each bar represents 100 infants. The numbers in the legends denote the scores of the item.

54. *Posture and movements of upper extremities while walking independently: presence of asymmetry (S)*

The presence of asymmetry in posture and movements of the upper extremities while walking independently is assessed (Video 7.9). The item can only be assessed in infants who are able to walk independently: that is, who obtained score 4 at item 51.

0 = cannot walk independently (item 51: score 1, 2, or 3)

1 = strong asymmetry, R/L worst side
2 = moderate asymmetry, R/L worst side
3 = no or mild asymmetry

Score 0   The infant cannot walk independently; the infant received score 1, 2, or 3 at item 51. Note that score 0 does not imply a worse score than score 1 or 2; it simply denotes that the score is not taken into account in the calculation of IMP scores.

Score 1   One upper extremity shows a clear stereotypy while the other upper extremity does not. For example, the arm is held in stereotyped shoulder abduction, elbow flexion, and fisting of the hand. The infant does not or only exceptionally shows other postures of the affected arm and hand: R=right and L=left.

Score 2   One upper extremity shows a moderate stereotypy while the other upper extremity does not. The moderate stereotypy may consist of a frequently occurring flexion of the elbow with or without abduction of the shoulder with or without fisting of the hand. The infant also shows other postures of the affected arm and hand: R=right and L=left.

Score 3   The infant shows no or a mild asymmetry in upper extremity posture while walking independently. The infant may occasionally show some asymmetry in elbow flexion/shoulder abduction.

55. *Variation in movements of arms and hands while walking independently (V)*

The size of the repertoire of arm and hand movements while walking independently is assessed. The repertoire of movements of both upper extremities is assessed (Video 7.10). This implies that the presence of a typical movement repertoire in one upper extremity in combination with a limited repertoire in the other upper extremity results in the classification 'insufficient variation'.

The item can only be assessed in infants who are able to walk independently: – that is, who obtained score 4 at item 51 – and who do not consistently hold their arms in high guard or semi-high guard (i.e., who obtained score 2 at item 53). In infants who occasionally show high- or semi-high-guard arm postures, only the repertoire of goal-directed arm movements is assessed.

   0 =   cannot walk independently (item 51: score 1, 2, or 3) or walks independently with arms consistently in high guard or semi-high guard (item 53: score 1)

   1 =   insufficient variation
   2 =   sufficient variation

Score 0   The infant cannot walk independently (received score 1, 2, or 3 at item 51) or is only able to walk independently with arms consistently held in high guard or semi-high guard (received score 1 at item 53). Note that score 0 does not imply a worse score than score 1 or 2; it simply denotes that the score is not taken into account in the calculation of IMP scores.

Score 1   The infant shows a limited repertoire of arm and hand movements consisting of a limited number of combinations of movements in the various joints of the upper extremities, with little variation in movement velocity and movement amplitude. Examples of stereotypes are an arm held in stereotyped shoulder abduction, elbow flexion, and fisting of the hand or the presence of repetitive, stereotyped, circular wrist movements or flapping arm movements.

Score 2   The infant shows various combinations of movements in the various joints of the upper extremities: for example, abduction and adduction movements, anteflexion and retroflexion movements, flexion, extension, and rotation.

56. Adaptability of movements of arms and hands while walking independently (A)

Adaptability of arm and hand movements while walking independently refers to the infant's ability to select efficient and goal-directed strategies from the repertoire of arm movements in each situation. The item can only be assessed in infants who are able to walk independently – that is, who received score 4 at item 51 – and who do not hold their arms consistently in high guard or semi-high guard: that is, who received score 2 at item 53.

> 0 = cannot walk independently (item 51: score 1, 2, or 3) or walks independently with arms consistently in high guard or semi-high guard (item 53: score 1)

Majority of movements:

1 = no selection
2 = adaptive selection

Score 0 The infant cannot walk independently (received score 1, 2, or 3 at item 51) or is only able to walk independently with arms consistently held in high guard or semi-high guard (received score 1 at item 53). Note that score 0 does not imply a worse score than score 1 or 2; it simply denotes that the score is not taken into account in the calculation of IMP scores.

Score 1 During the majority of walking sequences, the infant does not select efficient and goal-directed arm movements out of the repertoire of arm movements. He shows that he is exploring various upper extremity movements for either balancing or goal-directed activities of the arms and hands, but he does not or only occasionally selects an efficient strategy. Score 1 is also assigned if the infant has a motor repertoire which consists of only one strategy. Note that infants with semi-high-guard or high-guard posturing are assigned score 0.

Score 2 During the majority of walking sequences, the infant selects efficient and goal-directed arm movements out of the repertoire of arm movements. For instance, the infant is able to use his arms and hands in an efficient way to carry and manipulate toys while walking. A prerequisite for adaptive selection is that the repertoire consists of more than one motor strategy.

Figure 7.12 shows the development of adaptability in the movements of the arms and hands while walking independently in the norm population. Only a small proportion of infants who are able to walk independently without high-guard or semi-high-guard arm posture do not select adaptive arm movements during the majority of walking movements (1% to 4% of infants aged 11 to 18 months). The proportion of infants with efficient and goal-directed arm and hand movements while walking independently steadily increases with age, from 1% at 11 months to 48% at 15 months to 88% at 18 months.

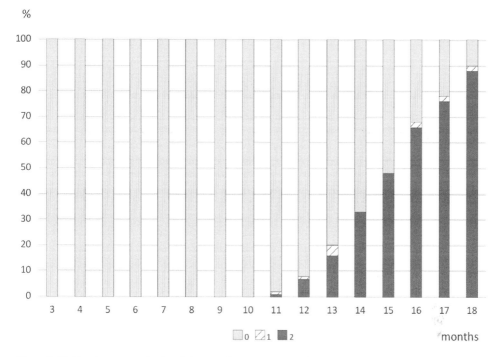

Figure 7.12 Development of adaptability of the movements of arms and hands during independent walking in the norm population (item 56). Each bar represents 100 infants. The numbers in the legends denote the scores of the item.

57. *Variation in trunk movements while standing and walking independently (V)*

The size of the repertoire of trunk movements while standing and walking independently is assessed. Trunk movements while standing and walking refers to the small movements used to vary and adjust posture while walking (Video 7.11). The item is only assessed in infants who are able to walk independently: that is, who achieved score 4 at item 51.

0 = cannot walk independently (item 51: score 1, 2, or 3)

1 = insufficient variation
2 = sufficient variation

Score 0   The infant cannot walk independently; the infant received score 1, 2, or 3 at item 51. Note that score 0 does not imply a worse score than score 1 or 2; it simply denotes that the score is not taken into account in the calculation of IMP scores.

Score 1   The infant shows a limited repertoire of trunk movements while standing and walking independently. For example, the infant has a prominent lordosis or keeps the entire trunk rigidly *en bloc* and does not show small adjustments in trunk posture while standing and walking.

Score 2   The infant shows a substantial repertoire of small movements of the trunk while standing and walking. Score 2 may also be assigned to infants with so-called toddling behaviour. Toddling is the characteristic walking pattern of novice walkers, consisting of a walking pattern with short, quick steps while the trunk shows more or less block-like movements (Hempel 1993, Hadders-Algra et al. 1998). Toddling does not, however, consist of a stereotyped and rigid trunk posture: that is, during toddling, small trunk movements are also present.

58.   *Adaptability of trunk movements while standing and walking independently (A)*

Adaptability of trunk movements while standing and walking independently refers to the infant's ability to select the most efficient trunk movements in each standing or walking situation (Video 7.12). The item is only assessed in infants who are able to walk independently: that is, who received score 4 at item 51.

  0 = cannot walk independently (item 51: score 1, 2, or 3)

  Majority of movements:

  1 = no selection
  2 = adaptive selection

Score 0   The infant cannot walk independently; the infant received score 1, 2 or 3 at item 51. Note that score 0 does not imply a worse score than score 1 or 2; it simply denotes that the score is not taken into account in the calculation of IMP scores.

Score 1   During the majority of standing and walking movements, the infant does not select efficient trunk movements. The movements reflect that the infant explores trunk movements to keep balance during standing and walking. Score 1 is also assigned if the infant has a motor repertoire which consists of only one strategy or if the infant shows consistent toddling. It may be argued that toddling is an adaptation of trunk behaviour by the novice walker to the insecure situation of learning to balance while walking: while toddling, the degrees of freedom in trunk movements are limited by contracting many postural muscles in the trunk (Hadders-Algra et al. 1998). Yet the toddling strategy precludes more subtle adjustments of trunk posture during walking. Therefore, toddling trunk movements are assigned score 1.

Score 2   During the majority of standing and walking movements, the infant is able to select the most efficient trunk movements. This means, for example, that the infant is able to adjust trunk movements efficiently in order to maintain balance while standing and walking. A prerequisite for adaptive selection is that the repertoire consists of more than one motor strategy.

  Figure 7.13 shows the development of adaptability of trunk movements while standing and walking independently in the norm population. The adaptability of trunk movements while standing and walking emerges at 11 months. This ability gradually increases with increasing age, from 2% at 11 months to 42% at 15 months to 89% at 18 months.

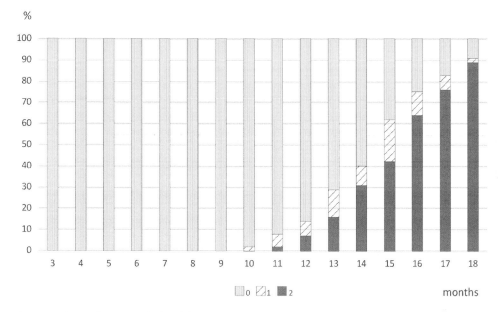

Figure 7.13 Development of adaptability of trunk movements while standing and independent walking in the norm population (item 58). Each bar represents 100 infants. The numbers in the legends denote the scores of the item.

59.   *Leg posture and movements while walking independently: presence of asymmetry (S)*

The presence of asymmetry in posture and movements of the legs while walking independently is assessed. Special attention is paid to the presence of moderate or marked stereotypes in the motor behaviour of one leg (Video 7.13). The item is only assessed in infants who are able to walk independently: that is, who received score 4 at item 51.

   0 = cannot walk independently (item 51: score 1, 2, or 3)

   1 = strong asymmetry, R/L worst side
   2 = moderate asymmetry, R/L worst side
   3 = no or mild asymmetry

Score 0   The infant cannot walk independently; the infant received score 1, 2, or 3 at item 51. Note that score 0 does not imply a worse score than score 1 to 3; it simply denotes that the score is not taken into account in the calculation of IMP scores.

Score 1   One leg shows a clear stereotypy (e.g., a clear plantar flexion of the foot or an extension-circumduction movement of the leg) while the other leg does not. The infant does not or only exceptionally shows other postures of the affected leg: R=right and L=left.

Score 2   One leg shows a moderate stereotypy while the other leg does not. In addition to the stereotypy, the affected leg also shows some other postures: R=right and L=left.

Score 3   The infant shows no or a mild asymmetry in leg posture while walking independently.

60.   *Variation in leg movements while walking independently (V)*

The size of the repertoire of leg movements while walking independently is assessed. It should be realized that the activity of walking itself limits the number of combinations of hip and knee movements. As a result, assessment of the repertoire of leg movements focuses on the presence of small variants. The repertoire of movements of both legs is assessed (Video 7.11). This implies that the presence of a typical movement repertoire in one leg in combination with a limited repertoire in the other leg results in the classification 'insufficient variation'. The item is only assessed in infants who are able to walk independently: that is, who received score 4 at item 51.

> 0 = cannot walk independently (item 51: score 1, 2, or 3)

> 1 = insufficient variation
> 2 = sufficient variation

Score 0   The infant cannot walk independently; the infant received score 1, 2, or 3 at item 51. Note that score 0 does not imply a worse score than score 1 or 2; it simply denotes that the score is not taken into account in the calculation of IMP scores.

Score 1   The infant shows a limited repertoire of leg movements while walking. This is reflected by the presence of stereotyped movements, such as extension-circumduction movements of the legs, stereotyped knee flexion, or consistently coming to a halt with hyperextended knees.

Score 2   The infant shows a substantial repertoire of walking strategies, which is reflected by the use of various combinations of movements in the various joints of the legs: for example, abduction and adduction movements, flexion, extension, and rotation.

61.   *Adaptability of leg movements while walking independently (A)*

Adaptability of leg movements while walking independently refers to the infant's ability to select the most efficient leg movements during each walking situation (Video 7.12). The item is only assessed in infants who are able to walk independently: that is, who received score 4 at item 51.

> 0 = cannot walk independently (item 51: score 1, 2, or 3)

> Majority of movements:

> 1 = no selection
> 2 = adaptive selection

Score 0   The infant cannot walk independently; the infant received score 1, 2, or 3 at item 51. Note that score 0 does not imply a worse score than score 1 or 2; it simply denotes that the score is not taken into account in the calculation of IMP scores.

Score 1   During the majority of walking sequences, the infant does not select efficient leg movements. Generally, the infant explores various leg movements, but the majority of the movements are not efficiently assisting the infant in maintaining balance. Score 1 is also assigned if the infant has a motor repertoire that consists of only one strategy.

Score 2   During the majority of walking sequences, the infant selects efficient leg movements that assist the infant in adapting his walking to varying situations (crossing the mattress, changing walking direction) and keeping balance. A prerequisite for adaptive selection is that the repertoire consists of more than one motor strategy.

Figure 7.14 shows the development of adaptability of leg movements while walking independently in the norm population. The adaptability of the leg movements while walking independently emerges at 11 to 13 months. Thereafter, the prevalence of adaptive leg movements gradually increases to 16% at 15 months and 66% at 18 months.

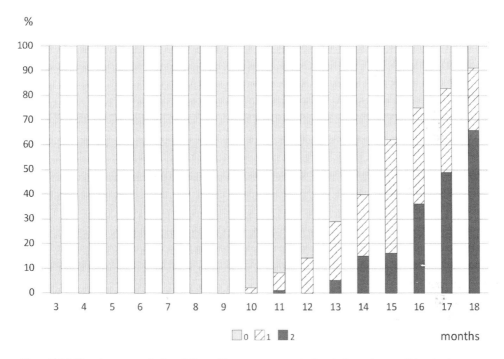

Figure 7.14 Development of adaptability of leg movements during independent walking in the norm population (item 61). Each bar represents 100 infants. The numbers in the legends denote the scores of the item.

62.   Heel-toe gait while walking independently (P)

Heel-toe gait refers to foot placement and lift while walking independently. Heel-toe gait is characterized by a marked heel strike well in front of the body with the toes lifted in the air, followed by toe contact and a subsequent heel lift during maintained toe contact in the end of the stance (Forssberg 1985, Lacquaniti et al. 2012, Video 7.14). The item is only assessed in infants who are able to walk independently: that is, who received score 4 at item 51.

Note that at the emergence of typical independent walking, the infant places his foot in a varied, virtually random way. After a couple of months of walking experience, the infant selects the heel-toe gait pattern increasingly often. Therefore, score 1 includes the occasional presence of a heel-toe gait pattern.

0 = cannot walk independently (item 51: score 1, 2, or 3)

1 = no or occasional heel-toe gait
2 = predominantly heel-toe gait

Score 0   The infant cannot walk independently; the infant received score 1, 2, or 3 at item 51. Note that score 0 does not imply a worse score than score 1 to 3; it simply denotes that the score is not taken into account in the calculation of IMP scores.

Score 1   The infant does not show heel-toe gait or only occasionally shows heel-toe gait but also shows many steps without a heel-toe sequence.
Score 2   The infant predominantly shows heel-toe gait while walking.

Figure 7.15 shows the development of heel-toe gait while walking independently in the norm population. The use of a predominant heel-toe gait pattern emerges at 16 months. At this age, 3% of infants use the heel-toe gait pattern predominantly. The prevalence of a predominant use of heel-toe gait rises to 11% at 18 months. This means that only a minority of infants in the age range of the IMP achieve the skill of a predominant use of the heel-toe gait pattern, turning item 62 into another 'difficult' IMP item.

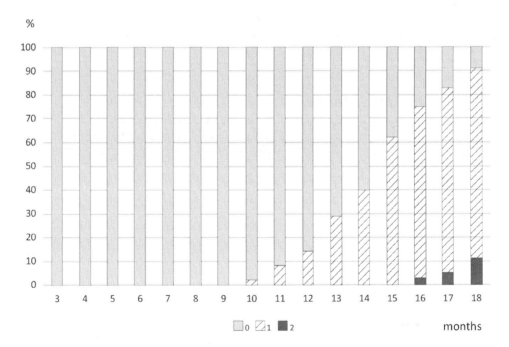

Figure 7.15 Development of heel-toe gait during independent walking in the norm population (item 62). Each bar represents 100 infants. The numbers in the legends denote the scores of the item.

63.   *Variation in foot movements while walking independently (V)*

The size of the repertoire of foot movements while walking independently is assessed (Video 7.11). The repertoire of movements of both feet is assessed. This implies that the presence of a typical movement repertoire in one foot in combination with a limited repertoire in the other foot results in the classification 'insufficient variation'. The form of the foot is not taken into account. The item is only assessed in infants who are able to walk independently: that is, who received score 4 at item 51.

0 = cannot walk independently (item 51: score 1, 2, or 3)

1 = insufficient variation
2 = sufficient variation

Score 0   The infant cannot walk independently; the infant received score 1, 2, or 3 at item 51. Note that score 0 does not imply a worse score than score 1 or 2; it simply denotes that the score is not taken into account in the calculation of IMP scores.

Score 1   The infant shows a limited repertoire of foot movements while walking, which is reflected by little variation in foot placement. Examples of stereo-typed foot movements while walking are clawing of toes, consistent exorota-tion or endorotation of the foot, and walking on tiptoes.

Score 2   The infant shows a substantial repertoire of foot movements while walking, which is reflected by a variation in foot placement and various movements in feet and toes.

64.   *Adaptability of foot movements while walking independently (A)*

Adaptability of foot movements during independent walking refers to the infant's ability to select the most efficient foot-placing movements during each walking situation (Video 7.12). The item is only assessed in infants who are able to walk independently: that is, who received score 4 at item 51.

0 = cannot walk independently (item 51: score 1, 2, or 3)

Majority of movements:

1 = no selection
2 = adaptive selection

Score 0   The infant cannot walk independently; the infant received score 1, 2, or 3 at item 51. Note that score 0 does not imply a worse score than score 1 or 2; it simply denotes that the score is not taken into account in the calculation of IMP scores.

Score 1   During the majority of walking sequences, the infant does not select efficient placement of the feet. Generally, the infant explores various ways of foot placement, but the majority of movements do not efficiently assist the infant in keeping balance, avoiding obstacles, or stepping on the mattress. Score 1 is also assigned if the infant has a motor repertoire that consists of only one stereotyped strategy.

Score 2   During the majority of walking sequences, the infant selects efficient placement of the feet. For example, the infant places his feet in such a way that he is able to avoid or step over objects on the floor. A prerequisite for adaptive selection is that the repertoire consists of more than one motor strategy.

Figure 7.16 shows the development of the adaptability of the feet while walking independently in the norm population. Adaptability of the feet while walking independently emerges at 14 or 15 months, when 1% to 2% of infants show this ability. The prevalence of adaptive foot movements while walking increases to 27% at 18 months. The developmental data of IMP's adaptability items of the trunk, legs and feet while walking independently show that, generally, the development of adaptive movements while walking follows a proximal-to-distal sequence.

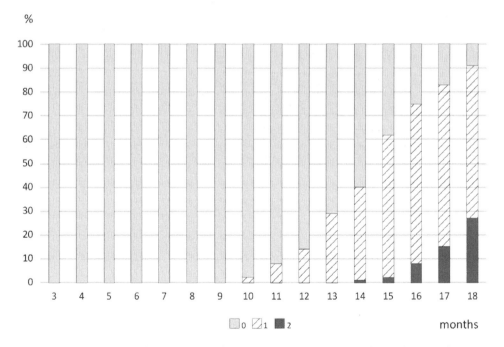

Figure 7.16 Development of adaptability of feet movements during independent walking in the norm population (item 64). Each bar represents 100 infants. The numbers in the legends denote the scores of the item.

65.   *Fluency of movements while walking independently (F)*

Fluency of motor behaviour denotes the presence of smooth, graceful movements without effort. Fluency in particular points to the velocity profile of movements. Fluent movements are characterized by gradual accelerations and decelerations (Hadders–Algra 2004, Video 7.15). The item is only assessed in infants who are able to walk independently: that is, who received score 4 at item 51.

0 = cannot walk independently (item 51: score 1, 2 or 3)

Majority of walking movements:

1 = non-fluent: stiff, jerky, floppy/sluggish, otherwise:
2 = fluent

Score 0   The infant cannot walk independently; the infant received score 1, 2, or 3 at item 51. Note that score 0 does not imply a worse score than score 1 or 2; it simply denotes that the score is not taken into account in the calculation of IMP scores.

Score 1   The majority of walking movements are non-fluent, indicating that they are not smooth, supple, or graceful. Various sorts of non-fluency can be distinguished, and an infant may show different types of non-fluent movements during a single assessment. Examples of non-fluent movements are stiff movements, jerky movements, and sluggish movements. Stiff movements lack ease of movement and have slow accelerations. Jerky movements denote the presence of sudden, abrupt movements with rapid acceleration. Floppy or sluggish movements are limp, torpid, and slow. If the non-fluent character of the movements cannot be described as stiff, jerky, or floppy/sluggish, the non-fluency is described with alternative, more appropriate words.

Score 2   The majority of walking movements have a fluent character, indicating that the movements are smooth, supple, and graceful.

8   Assessment of reaching, grasping, and manipulation of objects while sitting

This chapter contains the description of the IMP items assessed while reaching, grasping, and manipulating objects in a sitting position. Reaching, grasping, and manipulation in a sitting position are always assessed and always include a section during which the infant sits on the caregiver's lap. Additionally, reaching, grasping, and manipulation while sitting may be assessed while sitting independently.

Procedure

The standard procedure is that reaching, grasping, and manipulating objects while sitting is evaluated while the infant sits on the caregiver's lap, with the caregiver sitting on a chair or sofa (not on the floor). In general, this is performed as the last part of the IMP assessment. Care is taken that the infant sits comfortably in the midline of the caregiver's body (Figure 8.1). The caregiver does not receive specific instructions on the infant's postural support; the caregiver is only asked to ensure that the infant sits comfortably. For infants who are a bit shy or anxious, it may be better not to start the IMP assessment in a supine position, but rather on the caregiver's lap. Thus, the IMP assessment may also start with the evaluation of reaching, grasping, and manipulation while the infant sits on the caregiver's lap.

The examiner presents attractive small toys (about the size of the infant's hand) to the infant. First, one toy is presented to the infant. For infants with emerging reaching and grasping abilities, the toy is presented in the midline at arm's-length distance and kept there for a while. Arm's-length distance means not too far away and not too close to the body of the infant: for instance, not so close that an infant who produces prereaching movements directed towards the other hand in the midline might accidentally hit and grasp the toy. Pay close attention to the infant's visual attention. Repeat the toy presentation multiple times. When the infant is able to grasp the toy, allow him some time to manipulate the object. Next, the assessor retrieves the toy. Thereafter, a second toy is presented. Again, the infant is given ample time to find his own solution to get it. If the infant is able to handle two objects, the infant is offered two objects several times in succession. Next, the assessor evaluates whether the infant is able to grasp a third object while holding the other two. This would mean that the infant is able to hold two objects in one hand, implying that the infant is able to use the hand simultaneously as storage and a manipulative tool (Touwen 1976). Note that objects held in the mouth or objects held between hand and body are not considered 'objects held'. For the evaluation of reaching, grasping, and manipulation, it is important that the infant's face and eyes (visual attention) are also clearly recorded on video.

When the assessor has determined how many objects the infant can handle at a time (performance item 66), the focus of the assessment shifts to the evaluation of the variation

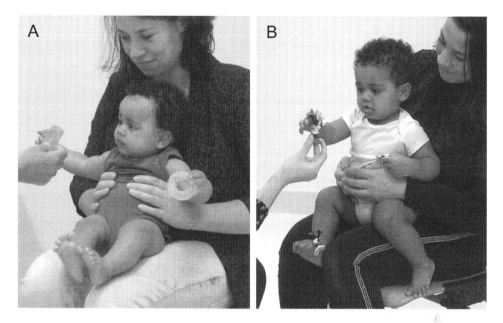

Figure 8.1 Evaluation of reaching, grasping, and manipulation while sitting on the caregiver's lap. The caregiver makes sure that infant sits comfortably. (A) Infant of six months; (B) infant of 12 months.

and adaptability of his arms and hands. To this end, the toys are presented one by one at a distance of about the length of the infant's arm (and not beyond!) at various positions in space. Several times, the object is also placed closer to the infant's body. The spatial variation is needed to assess the infant's repertoire of arm and hand movements (variation) and ability to adapt reaching movements to the specifics of the condition (adaptability). To assess variation and adaptability of hand and finger movements, a variety of toys with different shapes and sizes are used. First, simple rings are presented, followed by the presentation of more complex objects such as small puppets and small objects able to elicit a pincer grasp (e.g., the tip of a measuring tape; see also Figure 3.1 and Figure 8.6).

The reaching, grasping, and manipulative abilities of both arms and hands are evaluated. In case of an asymmetry in arm–hand performance, the severity of the asymmetry is evaluated by also presenting toys on the side of the worst performing arm and hand. The evaluation of the performance of reaching and grasping is based on the best performance observed; in case of asymmetric arm movements, this is based on the performance of the best arm and hand. Note that the asymmetry itself is scored at item 67.

In addition to the evaluation of reaching, grasping, and manipulation while sitting on the caregiver's lap, reaching, grasping, and manipulation may also be assessed when the infant sits independently on the floor or on the assessment mattress. The procedures are similar to those of the assessment of reaching, grasping, and manipulation while sitting on the caregiver's lap. Sitting independently is used especially for the evaluation of reaching, grasping, and manipulation in older infants, who sometimes prefer this situation to sitting on the caregiver's lap. If reaching, grasping, and manipulation are assessed not only on the caregiver's lap, but also while sitting independently on the floor or the assessment mattress, the scores of items 66 through 74 are based on the overall performance in both situations.

66.   *Reaching, grasping, and manipulation of objects (P)*

The infant's ability to reach, grasp, and manipulate objects while sitting is assessed (Video 8.1). The infant receives the score of the best performance even when this is achieved with only one hand.

> 1 = does not reach and does not show prereaching movements
> 2 = does not reach but shows prereaching movements
> 3 = reaches towards object but does not grasp it
> 4 = reaches towards, grasps, and holds object but does not manipulate object
> 5 = reaches towards, holds, and manipulates one object
> 6 = reaches towards, holds, and manipulates two objects
> 7 = reaches towards and holds ≥ three objects

Score 1   The infant does not reach towards the object and does not show prereaching movements (see score 2).

Score 2   The infant does not reach towards the object but shows prereaching movements. Prereaching movements are movements of arms, hands, and fingers in reaction to the presentation of an attractive object that do not result in an actual approach towards the object (Trevarthen 1984, Hadders-Algra 2018c). Examples of prereaching movements are mutual manipulation of hands, hand-mouth contact movements, and flapping abduction movements of the arms in response to the presentation of an attractive object (Video 8.1). To distinguish between spontaneous arm movements that are not related to the object presentation (score 1) and prereaching, close attention is paid to the infant's visual attention. Prereaching is associated with clear visual fixation of the object, which is often accompanied by a facial expression of vivid interest and movements of the mouth. In spontaneous, non–goal-directed movements of the arms, the infant does not pay visual attention to the object.

Score 3   The infant reaches towards the object, gets close to it, but does not grasp it. Reaching is defined as making a goal-directed movement with one or both arms towards the object (Touwen 1976). The hand may or may not touch the object (Video 8.1).

Score 4   The infant reaches towards, grasps, and holds the object. He does not manipulate the object within or between his hands, does not transfer the object from one hand to the other, and does not put the object into his mouth. Grasping is defined as approaching the object via a self-generated reaching movement with one or both hands, touching it, and getting hold of it. After grasping the object, the infant must hold the object for at least a few seconds to pass the item (Video 8.1). Note that the infant should grasp the object himself and that the object should not be put or pushed into the infant's hand by the examiner.

Score 5   The infant reaches towards, grasps, holds, and manipulates one object. Manipulation may consist, for example, of transferring the object to the other hand, moving the object within the hand, or putting the object into his mouth (Video 8.1). Infants who are able to grasp and hold two objects but who do not manipulate either object at all also are assigned score 5 (and not score 6).

Score 6   The infant holds one object and reaches towards a second object. This results in grasping of the second object, holding of the two objects, and some manipulation of at least one of the objects (Video 8.1). This also implies that infants who grasp a second object but immediately thereafter drop one of the objects are not assigned score 6.

Score 7   The infant holds two objects and reaches towards a third object. This results in grasping of the third object and holding all three objects (Figure 8.2, Video 8.1). Manipulation is not required to receive score 7; the focus of the item is on the ability to grasp an object with a hand that already holds another object. However, infants who grasp a third object but immediately thereafter drop one of the objects are not assigned score 7. Score 7 is also given when an infant is able to hold more than three objects.

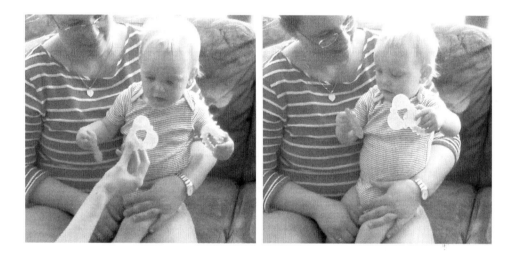

Figure 8.2 Infant of 14 months being able to reach towards and hold at least three objects (item 66)

Figure 8.3 shows the development of reaching, grasping, and manipulating objects in a sitting position in the norm population. At three months, 17% of infants do not show reaching attempts, 56% show prereaching movements, and only 1% are able to grasp and manipulate at least one object. At four months, 36% of the infants are able to grasp and manipulate at least one object, whereas at five months, 75% of infants have achieved this ability, with 35% being able to grasp and manipulate two objects. At six to eight months, the majority of infants (78% to 91%) are able to grasp and manipulate two objects, whereas 1% to 5% are able to handle three objects. From nine months onwards, the proportion of infants able to reach towards and get hold of at least three objects gradually increases from 15% at nine months to 40% to 47% at 11 to 13 months to about 80% at 16 to 18 months.

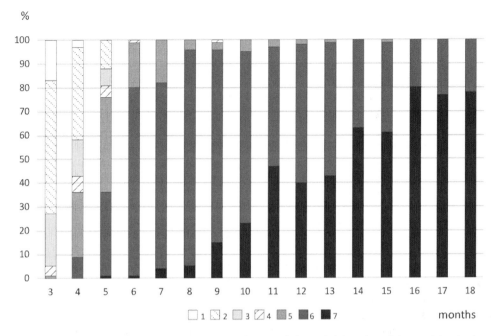

Figure 8.3 Development of reaching, grasping, and manipulation of objects in a sitting position in the norm population (item 66). Each bar represents 100 infants. The numbers in the legends denote the scores of the item.

67.   *Reaching, grasping, and manipulating objects: presence of asymmetry (S)*

The presence of asymmetry in arm and hand movements during (pre)reaching, grasping, and manipulation is assessed.

> 0 = the infant does not show prereaching or reaching movements (item 66: score 1)
>
> 1 = strong asymmetry, R/L worst side
> 2 = moderate asymmetry, R/L worst side
> 3 = no or mild asymmetry

Score 0   The infant does not show prereaching or reaching movements; the infant received score 1 at item 66. Therefore, the item cannot be assessed. Note that score 0 does not imply a worse score than score 1, 2, or 3; it simply denotes that the score is not taken into account in the calculation of IMP scores.

Score 1   A marked difference between right and left side is present in the posture and movements of the arm and/or hand during (pre)reaching, grasping, and manipulation. This means that the arm and hand on one side of the body show a stereotypy and only exceptionally show other postures or movements: R=right and L=left (Video 8.2).

Score 2 The infant shows a moderate asymmetry in his posture and movements of arm and/or hand during (pre)reaching, grasping, and manipulation, but both sides are involved in the goal-directed activities of arms and hands: R=right and L=left (Video 8.2).

Score 3 The infant shows no or only a mild asymmetry in his posture and movements of the hand or arm during (pre)reaching, grasping, and manipulation of objects. This means that a mild hand preference may be present (Videos 8.1 and 8.2).

68. *Variation in reaching movements of the arms (V)*

The size of the repertoire of movements of both arms is assessed (Video 8.3). This implies that the presence of a typical movement repertoire in one arm in combination with a limited repertoire in the other arm results in the classification 'insufficient variation'. If an infant shows a mix of reaching and prereaching movements, both reaches and prereaches are taken into account. Also, the repertoire of arm movements between the various reaching movements is taken into account in the evaluation of the variation in arm movements during the assessment of reaching. The repertoire of arm movements is not assessed when the infant only shows prereaching movements.

0 = the infant does not show reaching movements (item 66: score 1 or 2)

1 = insufficient variation
2 = sufficient variation

Score 0 The infant does not show reaching movements; the infant received score 1 or 2 at item 66. Therefore, the item cannot be assessed. Note that score 0 does not imply a worse score than score 1 or 2; it simply denotes that the score is not taken into account in the calculation of IMP scores.

Score 1 The infant shows a limited repertoire of reaching movements. The arm movements consist of a limited number of combinations of movements of the shoulder, elbow, and wrist (Figure 8.4). Examples of stereotyped patterns are simple extension movements, unilateral stereotyped flexion posturing, and stereotyped flapping or rotatory wrist movements occurring between the reaches.

Score 2 The infant shows reaching movements consisting of various combinations of movements of the shoulder (abduction, adduction, flexion, extension, endorotation, and exorotation), elbow (flexion, extension, pronation, supination) and wrist (flexion, extension, adduction, abduction) of both arms (Figure 8.4, Videos 8.1 and 8.3).

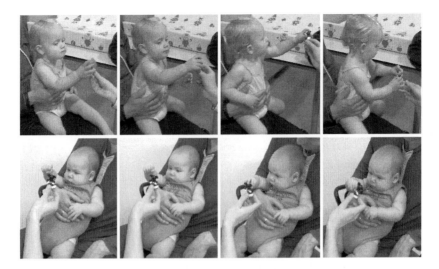

Figure 8.4 Variation in arm and hand movements during reaching, grasping, and manipulation in a sitting position (items 68 and 71). Upper panel: sufficient variation in arm and hand movements in infant of 14 months; lower panel: insufficient variation in arm and hand movements in infant of four months.

69. *Adaptability of reaching movements of the arms (A)*

Adaptability of reaching movements refers to the infant's ability to select the most appropriate and efficient reaching movement in each situation (Video 8.3).

0 = the infant does not show reaching movements (item 66: score 1 or 2)

Majority of movements:

1 = no selection
2 = adaptive selection

Score 0   The infant does not show reaching movements, and therefore, the item cannot be assessed. If an infant only shows prereaching movements, score 0 is also assigned. In other words, score 0 is assigned to infants who received score 1 or 2 at item 66. Note that score 0 does not imply a worse score than score 1 or 2; it simply denotes that the score is not taken into account in the calculation of IMP scores.

Score 1   During the majority of reaching movements, the infant does not select a specific, efficient reaching strategy out of the repertoire of reaching arm movements for specific situations. Score 1 is also assigned to infants with a motor repertoire which is limited to one strategy (Video 8.3).

Score 2   During the majority of reaching movements, the infant selects specific and efficient reaching strategies out of the repertoire of reaching strategies: that is, strategies that suit situations best (Video 8.3). A prerequisite for adaptive selection is the presence of a repertoire that consists of more than one motor strategy.

Figure 8.5 shows the development of adaptability of arm movements during reaching in the sitting position in the norm population. Adaptability of arm movements during reaching while sitting emerges at five months: 5% of the infants who are able to reach in a sitting position mostly show adaptive movements of the arm. The ability to mostly use adaptive reaching movements of the arms increases with increasing age: 50% of seven-month-olds and 94% of nine-month-olds have adaptive reaching movements of the arm in a sitting position. At 10 to 13 months, the prevalence of adaptive reaching movements of the arm is 97% to 99%. From 14 months onwards, all infants show adaptive movements of the arm while reaching in a sitting position.

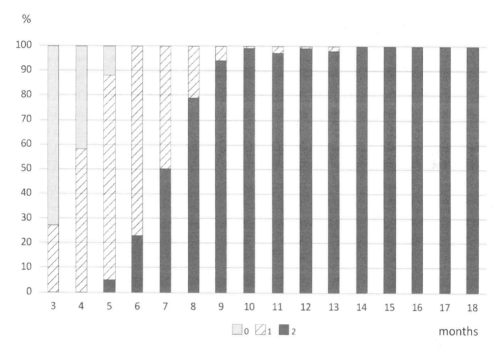

Figure 8.5 Development of adaptability of reaching movements of the arm in a sitting position in the norm population (item 69). Each bar represents 100 infants. The numbers in the legends denote the scores of the item.

70. *Type of grasping (P)*

The type of grasping is assessed during presentation of objects of various sizes, including small ones, and various forms to the infant. Grasping implies that the infant directs his hand via a self-produced movement to the object and gets hold of the object. In other words, manual behaviour elicited by the examiner putting an object directly into the infant's hand is not taken into account. Both hands are assessed separately, and the best performance of one of the hands is recorded.

Examples of toys which elicit the use of the inferior pincer grasp and pincer grasp are small pills, raisins, or mini-animals (5 × 5 mm). Care should be taken that the infant does not put small, non-edible objects into his mouth. A safe alternative is a retractable measuring tape that can be pulled out of its case (inferior pincer or pincer grasp) (see also Figure 3.1 and Figure 8.6).

0 = does not grasp object (item 66: score 1, 2, or 3)

1 = palmar grasp
2 = radial-palmar grasp or scissor grasp
3 = inferior pincer grasp
4 = pincer grasp

Score 0   The infant does not grasp objects, and therefore, the type of grasping cannot be assessed (item 66: score 1, 2, or 3). Note that score 0 does not imply a worse score than scores 1–4; it simply denotes that the score is not taken into account in the calculation of IMP scores.

Score 1   The infant shows palmar grasping: the infant uses the entire palmar surface of the hand and all fingers to grasp the object.

Score 2   The infant shows radial-palmar grasping or scissor grasping. In radial-palmar grasping, the infant mainly uses the radial half of his palm, including thumb and index finger, to grasp the object (Figure 8.6A; Touwen 1976). The scissor grasp means that the object is grasped between the volar surfaces of the extended thumb and index finger (Figure 8.6B; Touwen 1976).

Score 3   The infant uses the inferior pincer grasp: the object is grasped between the tip of the index finger and the volar side of the thumb; the index finger is flexed, and the thumb is extended (Figure 8.6C; Touwen 1976). In order to obtain score 4, the infant should not only place the fingers in the described manner, but also subsequently grasp the object.

Score 4   The infant uses the pincer grasp: the object is neatly grasped between the tips of index finger and thumb. Both index finger and thumb are flexed (Figure 8.6D; Touwen 1976). In order to obtain score 5, the infant should not only place the fingers in the described manner, but also subsequently grasp the object.

Note: it is sometimes difficult to see on the video whether the inferior pincer grasp or the pincer grasp is present. Therefore, we recommend that the assessor records the type of grasp observed during the 'real life' assessment. This is one of the two exceptions to the rule that the IMP assessment is based on a video recording of the infant's behaviour (the other being item 77).

Figure 8.7 shows the development of the type of grasping in the norm population. Infants aged three to four months who are able to grasp a toy virtually always use the palmar grasp. At five months, about a quarter of the infants who are able to grasp a toy use the radial-palmar grasp; the rest use the palmar grasp. Infants aged six to eight months mainly use the radial-palmar grasp, whereas the palmar grasp gradually disappears, and the inferior pincer grasp may be observed in some infants (1% to 4%). After the age of eight months, the prevalence of the inferior pincer grasp increases from 10% at nine months to 60% at 13 months. At 10 to 11 months a few infants (1% to 4%) show the pincer grasp. After the age of 11 months, the proportion of infants using the pincer grasp gradually increases from 18% at 12 months to 39% at 14 months to 64% to 69% of infants aged 16 to 18 months.

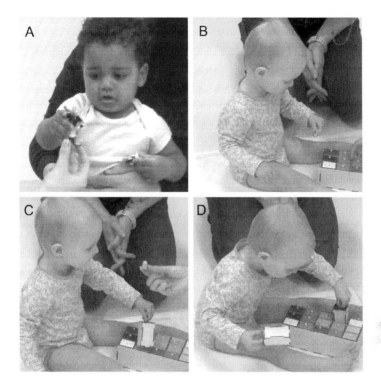

Figure 8.6 Type of grasping (item 70). (A) Radial–palmar grasp; (B) scissor grasp (extended index finger and extended thumb); (C) inferior pincer grasp (flexed index finger, extended thumb); (D) pincer grasp (flexed index finger and flexed thumb).

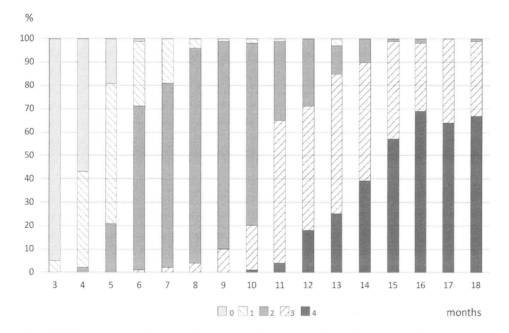

Figure 8.7 Development of the type of grasping in the norm population (item 70). Each bar represents 100 infants. The numbers in the legends denote the scores of the item.

71.   *Variation of hand movements while reaching, grasping, and manipulating (V)*

The size of the repertoire of movements of both hands is assessed (Video 8.4). This implies that the presence of a typical movement repertoire in one hand in combination with a limited repertoire in the other hand results in the classification 'insufficient variation'. Also, the repertoire of hand movements between the various reaching, grasping, and manipulative movements is taken into account in the evaluation of the variation in hand movements during the assessment of reaching. The repertoire of hand movements is not assessed when the infant only shows prereaching movements.

0 = the infant does not show reaching movements (item 66: score 1 or 2)

1 = insufficient variation
2 = sufficient variation

Score 0   The infant does not show reaching movements, and therefore, the item can-not be assessed; the infant received score 1 or 2 at item 66. Note that score 0 does not imply a worse score than score 1 or 2; it simply denotes that the score is not taken into account in the calculation of IMP scores.

Score 1   The infant shows only a limited number of ways of moving his hands dur-ing prereaching, reaching, grasping, and manipulation of objects. He shows a limited repertoire of hand and finger movements with little variation in the way in which the finger movements and positions are combined. Examples of stereotyped movement patterns are hand opening-closing movements in which the fingers move more or less synchronously with few independent finger movements and a consistent unilateral fisting posture (Figure 8.4, Video 8.4).

Score 2   The infant shows various ways to move his hands during prereaching, reaching, grasping, and manipulation of objects. He shows variation in the ways in which the finger movements and positions are combined (Figure 8.4, Video 8.4).

72.   *Adaptability of hand movements while reaching, grasping, and manipulating (A)*

Adaptability of hand movements refers to the infant's ability to select the most appropriate hand and finger movements in each situation. Adaptability of hand movements can be assessed when the hand approaches the object ('is the hand preshaped to the form and size of the object?'), during the actual grasping of the object, and during object manipulation.

0 = the infant does not show reaching movements (item 66: score 1 or 2)

Majority of movements:

1 = no selection
2 = adaptive selection

Score 0   The infant does not show reaching movements, and therefore, the item can-not be assessed; the infant received score 1 or 2 at item 66. Note that score 0 does not imply a worse score than score 1 or 2; it simply denotes that the score is not taken into account in the calculation of IMP scores.

Score 1   During the majority of reaching, grasping, and manipulative movements, the infant does not select a specific and efficient strategy out of the repertoire of grasping and/or manipulation strategies for specific situations (Video 8.4). Score 1 is also assigned to infants with a motor repertoire which is limited to one strategy.

Score 2   During the majority of reaching, grasping, and manipulative movements, the infant selects specific and efficient strategies out of the repertoire of grasping and/or manipulation strategies: that is, strategies that suit specific situations best (Video 8.4). Examples are preshaping of the hand to the form of the object in anticipation of the object grasp, the hands exhibiting efficient intra-manual object transfer, and a predominant and prompt selection of the inferior pincer grasp or pincer grasp when grasping a small object. A prerequisite for adaptive selection is the presence of a repertoire that consists of more than one motor strategy.

Figure 8.8 shows the development of the adaptability of hand movements during reaching, grasping, and manipulation in a sitting position in the norm population. Adaptability of hand movements emerges at eight to ten months, when 1% to 3% of infants show adaptive hand movements. After the age of ten months, the prevalence of adaptive hand movements gradually increases with increasing age, from 13% at 11 months to 57% at 14 months to 80% at 16 months to 85% to 89% at 17 to 18 months. This means that the development of adaptability in the movements of the upper extremities – like that in the lower extremities – generally follows a proximal-to-distal sequence.

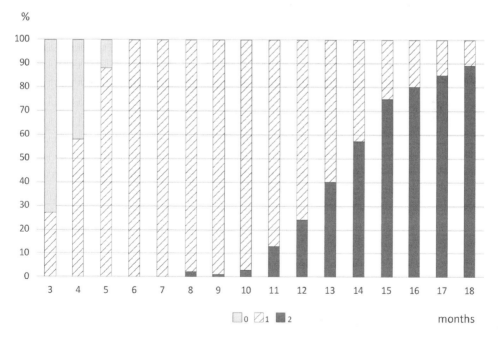

Figure 8.8 Development of adaptability of hand movements during reaching, grasping, and manipulation in a sitting position in the norm population (item 72). Each bar represents 100 infants. The numbers in the legends denote the scores of the item.

73.   Tremor during prereaching and reaching (F)

A tremor is an involuntary, oscillating movement with a fixed frequency (Piña-Garza and James 2019). Two types of tremors can be distinguished: the most frequently occurring type is a tremor with high frequency (≥6/sec) and low amplitude (≤3 cm). The other, less often observed type is a tremor with low frequency (>6/sec) and high amplitude (>3 cm) (Touwen 1976). At this item tremors superimposed on reaching or prereaching movements are assessed. Note that irregular, zig-zag movements are not regarded as tremor.

0 = the infant does not show prereaching or reaching movements (item 66: score 1)

1 = frequently present, describe type:
2 = not or occasionally present

Score 0   The infant does not show prereaching or reaching movements; the infant received score 1 at item 66. Therefore, the item cannot be assessed. Note that score 0 does not imply a worse score than score 1 or 2; it simply denotes that the score is not taken into account in the calculation of IMP scores.

Score 1   The infant shows tremors during the majority of prereaching, reaching, grasping, and manipulative movements (Video 8.5). Describe the type of tremor. The most commonly observed tremors are tremors with a high frequency (≥6/sec) and a low amplitude (≤3 cm) and those with a low frequency (<6/sec) and a high amplitude (>3 cm).

Score 2   The infant does not or only occasionally shows a tremor during prereaching, reaching, grasping, and manipulative movements (Video 8.5). Tremor may be present during some of the prereaching, reaching, grasping, and manipulative movements, but during the majority of arm and hand movements, tremor is absent.

74.   Fluency of movements during prereaching and reaching (F)

Fluency of motor behaviour denotes the presence of smooth, graceful movements without effort. Fluency in particular points to the velocity profile of movements. Fluent movements are characterized by gradual accelerations and decelerations (Hadders-Algra 2004).

0 = the infant does not show prereaching or reaching movements (item 66: score 1)

Majority of movements:

1 = non-fluent: stiff, jerky, floppy/sluggish, otherwise:
2 = fluent

Score 0   The infant does not show prereaching or reaching movements; the infant received score 1 at item 66. Therefore, the item cannot be assessed. Note that score 0 does not imply a worse score than score 1 or 2; it simply denotes that the score is not taken into account in the calculation of IMP scores.

Score 1   The majority of the prereaching, reaching, grasping, and manipulative move-ments are non-fluent, indicating that they are not smooth, supple, or graceful (Video 8.5). Various sorts of non-fluency can be distinguished, and an infant may show different types of non-fluent movements during a single assessment. Examples of non-fluent movements are stiff movements, jerky movements, and sluggish movements. Stiff movements lack ease of movement and give the impression of resistance. Jerky movements denote the presence of sudden, abrupt movements. Floppy or sluggish movements are limp, torpid, and slow. If the non-fluent character of the movements cannot be described as stiff, jerky, or floppy/sluggish, describe the non-fluency in alternative, more appro-priate words.

Score 2   The majority of the prereaching, reaching, grasping, and manipulative move-ments have a fluent character, indicating that the movements are smooth, supple, and graceful (Video 8.5).

9   General

Items observed throughout the assessment

This chapter contains the description of the IMP items that are assessed during the entire IMP assessment.

75.   Variation in facial expression (V)

Variation in facial expression denotes the presence of a repertoire of facial expressions. Humans, like great apes but unlike monkeys, have a large repertoire of facial expressions (De Waal 2003) generated by a complex facial muscular system (Cattaneo and Pavesi 2014).

    1 = insufficient variation
    2 = sufficient variation

Score 1   The infant shows a limited repertoire of facial expressions (Figure 9.1).
Score 2   The infant shows a substantial repertoire of facial expressions. The facial expressions are brought about by muscle activity in various parts of the face, such as the muscles around the eyes and the mouth, and are characterized by various combinations of muscle activity in these regions (Figure 9.1).

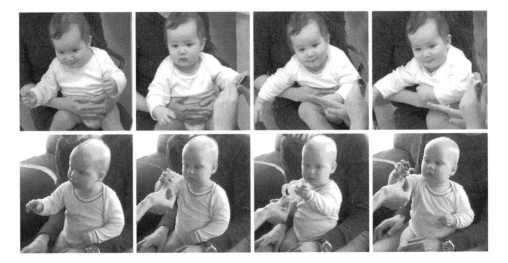

Figure 9.1 Variation in facial expression (item 75). Upper panel: infant with sufficient variation in facial expression; lower panel: infant with insufficient variation in facial expression.

76.   *Adaptability of facial expression (A)*

Adaptability of facial expression refers to the infant's ability to select the most appropriate facial expression in each situation.

Majority of movements:

1 = no selection
2 = adaptive selection

Score 1   Most of the time, the infant does not select specific facial expressions for specific situations out of the repertoire of facial expressions. This means that it is difficult for the observer to read in the infant's face what the infant's intentions and emotions are. Score 1 is also assigned if the infant has a facial expression repertoire which consists of a single, usually bland expression.

Score 2   Most of the time, the infant selects specific facial expressions for specific situations. This means that it is relatively easy to understand the infant's intentions and emotions. A prerequisite for adaptive selection is that the repertoire consists of more than one expression.

77.   *Drooling (V)*

Drooling is the clearly visible spilling of saliva from the mouth (McInerney et al. 2019). Typically developing infants may show some drooling when they explore an object with their mouths. Drooling is included in the domain of variation as marked drooling reflects the presence of stereotyped orofacial movements.

1 = marked drooling
2 = no or little drooling

Score 1   The infant shows marked drooling. This is, for instance, reflected by large wet spots on the infant's clothes (Figure 9.2).

Score 2   The infant does not drool or shows only occasional drooling during the assessment.

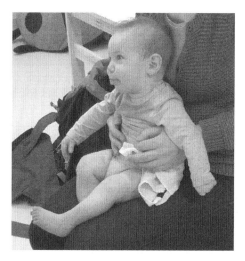

Figure 9.2 Marked drooling reflected by the large wet spot on the infant's clothes (item 77)

Note: it is sometimes difficult to see on the video whether the infant shows marked drooling or not. Therefore, we recommend that the assessor records the presence of marked drooling during the 'real life' assessment. This is one of the two exceptions to the rule that the IMP assessment is based on a video recording of the infant's behaviour (the other being the presence of the inferior pincer grasp or pincer grasp at item 70).

78.   *Presence of stereotyped tongue protrusion (V)*

Stereotyped tongue protrusion denotes the presence of either repetitive tongue protrusion movements with the tongue appearing between the lips about every two seconds (Hadders-Algra et al. 1997) or often-occurring periods during which the tongue protrudes between the lips (Video 9.1).

    1 = yes
    2 = no

Score 1   Yes, the infant shows stereotyped tongue protrusion.
Score 2   No, the infant does not show stereotyped tongue protrusion.

79.   *Tremor (F)*

A tremor is an involuntary, oscillating movement with a fixed frequency (Piña-Garza and James 2019). Two types of tremors can be distinguished: the most frequently occurring type is a tremor with a high frequency (≥6/sec) and a low amplitude (≤3 cm). The other, less-often-observed type is a tremor with a low frequency (<6/sec) and a high amplitude (>3 cm) (Touwen 1976).

   At this item only tremors observed during spontaneous motor behaviour in supine, prone, sitting, standing, and walking positions are assessed. The presence of tremors superimposed on prereaching and reaching movements are recorded separately (items 20 and 73).

    1 = frequently present, describe type:
    2 = not or occasionally present

Score 1   The infant frequently shows a tremor during spontaneous motor behaviour. Describe the type of tremor. The most commonly observed tremors are tremors with a high frequency (≥6/sec) and a low amplitude (≤3 cm) and those with a low frequency (<6/sec) and a high amplitude (>3 cm).
Score 2   The infant does not or only occasionally shows a tremor during spontaneous motor behaviour.

80.   *Fluency of motor behaviour (F)*

Fluency of motor behaviour denotes the presence of smooth, graceful movements without effort. Fluency in particular points to the velocity profile of movements. Fluent movements are characterized by gradual accelerations and decelerations (Hadders-Algra 2004).

   At this item, the overall impression on fluency of motor behaviour during the assessment in supine, prone, sitting, standing, and walking positions is assessed. The fluency of reaching behaviour in supine and sitting positions is not taken into account at this item; this is recorded separately (item 74 and, in part, item 21).

Majority of movements:

1 = non-fluent: stiff, jerky, floppy/sluggish, otherwise:
2 = fluent

Score 1   The majority of the movements are non-fluent, indicating that they are not smooth, supple, or graceful. This means that movements are non-fluent in most of the conditions assessed: for instance, when an infant is assessed in three conditions, such as in supine, prone, and sitting positions, fluency is given score 1 if the movements are non-fluent in two of the three conditions. Various sorts of non-fluency can be distinguished, and an infant may show different types of non-fluent movements during a single assessment. Examples of non-fluent movements are stiff movements, jerky movements, and sluggish movements. Stiff movements lack ease of movement and give the impression of resistance. Jerky movements denote the presence of sudden, abrupt movements. Floppy or sluggish movements are limp, torpid and slow. If the non-fluent character of the movements cannot be described as stiff, jerky, or floppy/sluggish, describe the non-fluency in alternative, more appropriate words.

Score 2   The majority of the movements have a fluent character, indicating that the movements are smooth, supple, and graceful. This means that movements are fluent in most of the conditions assessed: for instance, when an infant is assessed in three conditions, such as while prone, while sitting, and while standing and walking, fluency is alluded score 2 if the movements are fluent in two of the three conditions.

10 Clinical application and significance of the IMP

The IMP has been designed as an instrument to evaluate motor behaviour in infants and young children up to and including the age of walking independently for a couple of months. It is a reliable measurement with adequate validity. Moreover, it has a good responsiveness to change related to early intervention (Chapter 3). The IMP has two goals: (1) to monitor infant motor development or – phrased more specifically – to follow infant development in the IMP domains of variation, adaptability, symmetry, fluency, and performance and (2) to detect infants at high risk of developmental disorders. The IMP is especially useful in groups of at-risk infants, such as preterm infants or infants with complex congenital heart disease, not just because it facilitates the detection of infants at high risk of developmental disorders, but even more because it furnishes directions for early intervention.

In the following sections, we discuss the significance of low scores in the five IMP domains. Each section starts with the presentation of the IMP-percentile values based on the Dutch norm reference group of 1,700 infants aged 2 to 18 months (see Chapter 3).[1] The statistical background of the computation of the percentile curves is explained in Box 10.1. Next, the clinical application of the IMP is illustrated by a further discussion of the two clinical examples introduced in Chapter 1 (Box 10.2). Concluding remarks complete the chapter.

Box 10.1 Computation of IMP percentile curves

In preparation for the construction of the age-specific reference values (percentile curves) of the IMP, we investigated the performance of various statistical methods through a series of simulation studies using this particular type of data, especially with regard to different sample sizes (e.g., adaptability data are not available for all infants).

For the total IMP score and the adaptability domain scores, we used the LMS method, a semi-parametric approach where mean, standard deviation, and skewness are modelled as functions of age and fitted with cubic splines and where data are Box-Cox transformed to resemble the normal distribution, using R version 3.6.1. and R package GAMLSS (Rigby and Stasinopoulos

---

1 Note that the age of two months was included for statistical reasons. The lowest age for which the IMP has been validated is three months.

2005, R Core Team 2019). For the age-dependent performance domain (non-parametric) quantile-regression based models, again, using cubic splines proved to be the best choice.

We created age-specific reference values for the total IMP score and for the performance and adaptability domains, using the cross-sectional data set consisting of the IMP scores of the infants of the Dutch IMP-SINDA norm reference study. We present percentile curves for the 15%, 50%, and 85% percentiles for all three scores (total IMP scores and the performance and adaptability scores), as well as additional 5% curves for the total IMP scores and performance domain scores. Model fit was checked by comparing the expected with the actual observed percentage of cases below each percentile, as well as by examining worm plots and Q statistics for the fitted LMS models.

Variation domain

The IMP variation domain is a novel motor domain rooted in the NGST (Chapter 2). It describes a fundamental aspect of infant motor behaviour. The variation domain is not age-dependent (Heineman et al. 2008). Hence, we calculated age-independent percentile values (Table 10.1). The values indicate that the large majority of infants of the general population have a varied repertoire: half of the infants have a variation score of 95%. This implies that these infants only show insufficient variation in the movements described by one or two of the variation items, whereas the movements described in the rest of the variation items manifest sufficient variation. This corresponds to the notion that only a significantly reduced variation is a marker of brain dysfunction: that is, signals impaired subcortical-cortical connectivity (an impairment in the 'hardware' of the brain) (Hadders-Algra 2010, 2018b; Chapter 2). The presence of a low variation score indicates a high risk of a developmental disorder, in particular CP. Yet it should be realized that the variation score in young infants who have been critically ill in the neonatal period – for instance, infants born very preterm (before 32 weeks of gestation) or with a complex congenital heart disease – may also be lower because of limited movement experiences during neonatal illness (Hadders-Algra 2021c). Illness reduces the drive for movement exploration, and its accompanying disuse is associated with a moderate reduction of variation (Bos et al. 1997). Also, in infants with unilateral CP, disuse of the most affected side may aggravate the reduced variation brought about by the brain lesion (Hadders-Algra 2021c; see the section on the symmetry that follows). This implies that a low variation score invokes the need of further diagnostics, requests a longitudinal monitoring of the infant's development, and indicates a need for early intervention.

For early intervention, a low variation score means that caregivers need to be informed that the infant may profit from being exposed to varied situations during daily caregiving activities (Dirks et al. 2011, Akhbari Ziegler et al. 2019). For instance, caregivers may carry the infant in various ways, they may dress the infant in varied positions (e.g., supine or sitting), or with varied approaches (e.g., laterally or frontally), or they may play with

Table 10.1 Percentile values for the scores of the IMP variation, symmetry, and fluency domains

IMP domain	P5	P15	P50	P85
Variation	82	88	95	100
Symmetry				
Infants <6 months	75	83	95	100
Infants ≥6 months	95	100	100	100
Fluency	70	75	90	100

P5=5th percentile, P15=15th percentile, P50=50th percentile, P85=85th percentile

the infant with a variety of toys in a variety of positions (e.g., supine, semi-reclined, sitting in a chair or on a lap, or prone).

Research has demonstrated that exposing low-risk infants born very preterm to ample varying experiences in daily life is associated with improved variation scores: that is, an increase in the infant's movement repertoire (Sgandurra et al. 2016, 2017, Akhbari Ziegler et al. 2020). Presumably, the initial reduction of the movement repertoire in these infants is based on the limited experience in the neonatal period and not on the presence of a significant lesion of the brain. Studies of infants at very high risk of CP (Hielkema et al. 2011, 2020) indicate, however, that early intervention with ample varying experiences in daily life does not result in an enlargement of the movement repertoire in these infants; the infants' variation scores remain low. Many of the studied infants had a significant lesion of the brain, such as periventricular leukomalacia or a cortical infarction. This underlines the notion that serious reductions in variation are markers of a structural impairment of the brain.

In infants who continue to have very low variation scores, the risk of being diagnosed with CP is very high. Infants who show a very limited movement repertoire throughout infancy run a high risk of contractures and deformities due to the continuous presence of stereotyped movements and postures. For these infants, a major aim of early intervention is to prevent contractures and deformities. This is primarily achieved by means of the introduction at an early age of sitting, lying and, standing devices (Thunberg et al. 2021). In addition, it is conceivable that exposing these infants to varied challenges that elicit self-generated movements may assist in the prevention of contractures and deformities (Novak et al. 2020).

Adaptability domain

The IMP adaptability domain is the other novel domain based on the NGST. Adaptability scores can be calculated in infants older than six months. Before that age, adaptability is only present to a limited extent; it is first from six months onwards that adaptability starts to bloom (Heineman et al. 2010b). The adaptability scores are clearly age dependent (Heineman et al. 2008). This means that infants with increasing age and increasing experience are better able to adapt their movements efficiently to the specifics of the situation. Figure 10.1 presents the percentile curves of the

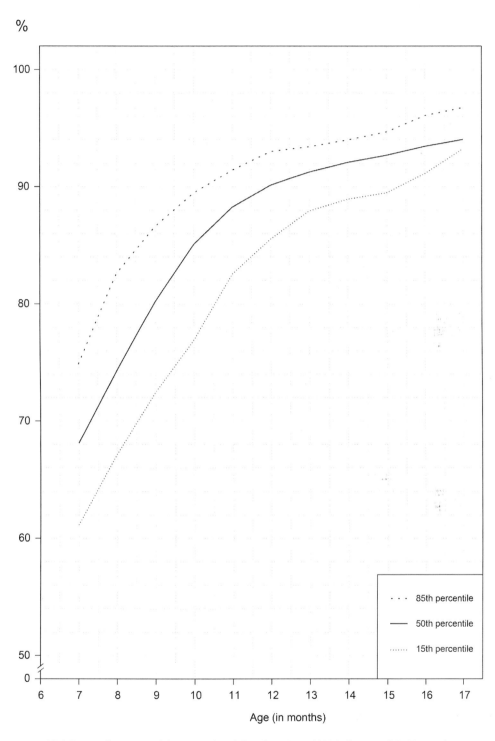

Figure 10.1 Percentile curves of the IMP adaptability domain in 1100 infants aged 7–17 months

Table 10.2 Age-dependent percentile values for the adaptability domain scores

Age in months	P15	P50	P85
7	61	68	75
8	67	74	82
9	72	80	87
10	77	85	89
11	82	88	91
12	86	90	93
13	88	91	93
14	89	92	94
15	91	93	95
16	93	93	96
17	94	94	97

P15=15th percentile, P50=50th percentile, P85=85th percentile

Values of 18 months are not provided, as the top end (highest age category) of the adaptability domain could not be modelled reliably due to lack of score variation in the data (see Figure 10.1).

adaptability scores of the infants in the Dutch norm reference group. Table 10.2 provides the numerical details.

Reduced adaptability may be the result of a lesion of the brain (an impairment in the 'hardware' of the brain), but more often, it is associated with altered settings of neurotransmitter systems: for instance the monoaminergic systems (an impairment in the 'software' of the brain; see Chapter 2). The altered neurotransmitter settings may have a genetic origin – for instance, in children with Attention-Deficit/Hyperactivity Disorder (ADHD) (Bonvicini et al. 2018) – or may be the result of stress in early life. Stress in early life may involve physiological and/or psychological stress. Examples of stress in early life are being born preterm – especially when it results in an admission to the neonatal intensive care unit – intrauterine growth retardation, and maternal stress during pregnancy (Braun et al. 2017, Hadders-Algra 2021d).

Lower adaptability scores are associated with lower intelligence quotient scores at school age (Wu et al. 2020b). This confirms the idea that adaptability scores reflect the infant's capacity to explore movements, to discover the world, and to learn from trial-and-error experiences. It is well known that children with developmental motor disorders, such as CP and DCD, have impaired motor learning (Prado et al. 2017, Wilson et al. 2017). They need more trial-and-error experiences than typically developing children in order to build motor reference frameworks allowing for an immediate and prompt selection of the most efficient movement in each specific situation. In other words, they need more movement experience than typically developing children before they achieve the ability of automatic, feedforward, anticipatory movement control (Chapter 2; Hadders-Algra et al. 1999).

For early intervention, this means that infants with reduced adaptability will profit from ample experience of self-generated movements allowing for ample trial and error: that is, self-generated movement feedback (Hadders-Algra 2021c). It implies that caregivers need to receive information on which activities the infant is about to master. This allows caregivers to understand which activities they may integrate into daily caregiving activities. Health professionals may provide caregivers with hints and suggestions on how to do this and how to playfully challenge the infant to perform new motor activities. This is one of the elements of the family-centred intervention programme COPing with and CAring for Infants with Special Needs (COPCA) (Dirks et al. 2011, Akhbari Ziegler et al. 2019). An early intervention study on COPCA demonstrated that coaching families to implement these strategies was associated with significant improvements in the adaptability scores (Hielkema et al. 2011).

Symmetry domain

The IMP symmetry domain describes a classical aspect of infant motor behaviour. The data of the Dutch norm reference group illustrate that mild-to-moderate asymmetries in motor behaviour occur especially in young infants; from six months onwards, the prevalence of asymmetries is very low. These findings correspond to the notion that young infants often show a head position preference to one side: an asymmetry that is often shown in more than one position. This positional preference is virtually gone when infants have reached the age of six months (Straathof et al. 2020). Due to the prevalence of different asymmetries in infants younger than six months and infants aged 6 to 18 months, the two age groups have different percentile values (Table 10.1).

At any age, low symmetry scores, reflecting a consistent asymmetry in multiple parts of the body, have clinical significance. They may be a marker of neurological dysfunction, including unilateral CP, especially when the asymmetries emerge in early infancy and continue to be present after the age of five months (Sakzewski et al. 2019, Wu et al. 2020b). The consistent asymmetries require further diagnostics and early intervention.

Early intervention in infants with asymmetries involves making caregivers aware of how they can challenge the child to use both sides of the body equally often. In young infants with a head position preference, caregiver guidance focuses on provision of information on environmental stimuli (taking care that the interesting environment – e.g., light, colourful objects, people – is at the infant's non-preferred side), positioning the infant (creating variation in infant position during, e.g., feeding and carrying), and promoting play in the prone position. (For more details, see Hadders-Algra 2021d.) In infants with or at high risk of unilateral CP who manifest especially with a consistent asymmetry in upper-limb function, early intervention aims at providing the caregivers with information on how they can promote symmetric upper-limb activities. To this end, the baby variant of constraint-induced movement therapy (baby-CIMT) may be applied (Eliasson et al. 2018), but intensive bilateral arm movement training is equally effective in promoting mobility in both arms and hands (Chamudot et al. 2018). Presumably, the positive effect of these intervention approaches may be attributed mainly, but not exclusively, to the counteraction of the disuse component of the reduced variation and asymmetry (Sterling et al. 2013, Kwon et al. 2014, Manning et al. 2016).

Fluency domain

The IMP fluency domain furnishes information on a classical aspect of infant motor behaviour: it supplies information on how well the infant is able to modulate movement accelerations and decelerations. The presence of non-fluent movements is not age dependent. Hence, we calculated age-independent percentile values (Table 10.1). The values indicate that about half the infants of the general population manifest non-fluency in part of their movements. In other words, many typically developing infants do not move perfectly fluently.

Fluency is a movement aspect that is sensitive to minor alterations in neural function. Cases in point are the non-fluent movements of crying babies (Hadders-Algra 2004) and the non-fluent movements of adults induced by nervousness or fatigue after intensive physical exercise (Growdon et al. 2000). The sensitivity of movement fluency to minor alterations in neural setting has turned fluency scores into sensitive instruments to evaluate subtle effects of environmental conditions in early life. An example is the association of breastfeeding with a higher prevalence of fluent movements at 3 and 18 months (Huisman et al. 1995, Bouwstra et al. 2003).

Most infants with non-fluent movements show jerky movements or a mix of jerky and stiff movements (Groen et al. 2005). Consistently stiff movements are relatively uncommon. Consistently stiff movements in combination with a marked reduction of variation have been associated with a high risk of CP (Groen et al. 2005, Hamer et al. 2011).

Non-fluent movements easily catch the attention of caregivers and professionals. Yet their clinical significance is very limited. Therefore, this aspect of infant motor behaviour does not require specific attention during early intervention. The focus of early physiotherapeutic intervention is on enabling mobility: that is, promoting the infant's abilities to maintain and change body position; to move around; and to carry, move, and handle objects. This may be achieved by provision of ample, varied, and challenging experiences of self-generated movements (Hadders-Algra 2021c). A potential positive side effect of being able to achieve certain motor abilities with less effort may be an increase in movement fluency.

Performance domain

The IMP performance domain is the only domain of the IMP that does not evaluate an aspect of movement quality. The performance domain measures what the infant is able to achieve in terms of motor abilities. The performance scores are strongly age dependent (Heineman et al. 2008). With increasing age and increasing experience, infants master increasingly more motor skills. Figure 10.2 presents the percentile curves of the performance scores of the infants of the Dutch norm reference group. Table 10.3 provides the numerical details. The data show that the majority of 18-month-old infants do not achieve the maximum score of 100%; only 15% of 18-month-olds score 97% or more.

A low performance score indicates that the infant is relatively slow in the achievement of multiple motor milestones. A delay in multiple milestones is – in contrast to a delay in a single milestone – a well-known biomarker of developmental disorders (Hadders-Algra 2021a). Low performance scores are associated with an increased risk of CP (Heineman et al. 2011) and lower intelligence quotients at school age (Wu et al. 2020b). A low performance score invokes the need of further diagnostics, longitudinal monitoring of development, and early intervention.

In early intervention, the performance domain is an excellent tool to determine short-term goals of intervention. Caregivers who attend the IMP assessment will notice which skills the infant has achieved and which abilities the infant presumably will be able to master in the near future. This awareness arises especially when health professionals explain to the caregivers what the infant is doing during the assessment. Knowledge about the motor skills which the infant is about to master allows caregivers to discuss with health professionals how practise of the emerging skills may be integrated into daily caregiving

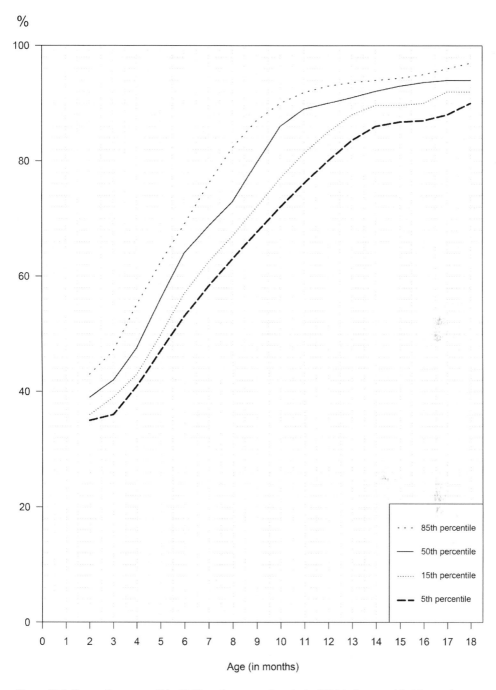

Figure 10.2 Percentile curves of the IMP performance domain in 1700 infants aged 2–18 months

Table 10.3 Age-dependent percentile values for the performance domain scores

Age in months	P5	P15	P50	P85
3	36	39	42	47
4	41	43	48	55
5	47	50	56	62
6	53	57	64	69
7	58	62	69	76
8	63	67	73	82
9	68	72	80	87
10	72	77	86	90
11	76	81	89	92
12	80	85	90	93
13	84	88	91	94
14	86	90	93	94
15	87	90	94	95
16	87	90	94	95
17	88	92	94	96
18	90	92	94	97

P5=5th percentile, P15=15th percentile, P50=50th percentile, P85=85th percentile

activities. Integration into daily caregiving activities is a practical means to achieve a high dosage of practise (Dirks et al. 2016). High dosage is a crucial element in the success of early intervention, but if it is perceived as frequent therapy, it is associated with a high burden for caregivers (Hadders-Algra 2021c).

Total IMP score

The total IMP score summarizes – or rather, averages – the scores of the IMP domains. In infants aged six months and younger, the total IMP score is based on the average of four domains (variation, symmetry, fluency, and performance); in infants aged more than six months, it is based on all five IMP domains. Due to the clear age dependency of the adaptability and performance domains, the total IMP score is also strongly age dependent (Heineman et al. 2008, 2010a). Figure 10.3 presents the percentile curves of the total IMP scores of the infants of the Dutch norm reference group. Tables 10.4 and 10.5 provide the numerical details.

A low total IMP score signals high risk of a developmental disorder, including CP (Heineman et al. 2011). It is also associated with a lower intelligence quotient at pre-school and school age (Heineman et al. 2018, Wu et al. 2020b). This means that a low total IMP score warrants further diagnostics, longitudinal monitoring of infant development, and early intervention. The total IMP score does not provide specific clues for intervention. The quintessence of the IMP for early intervention is furnished by the profile of the scores in the various domains. Table 10.6 summarizes the suggestions for early intervention.

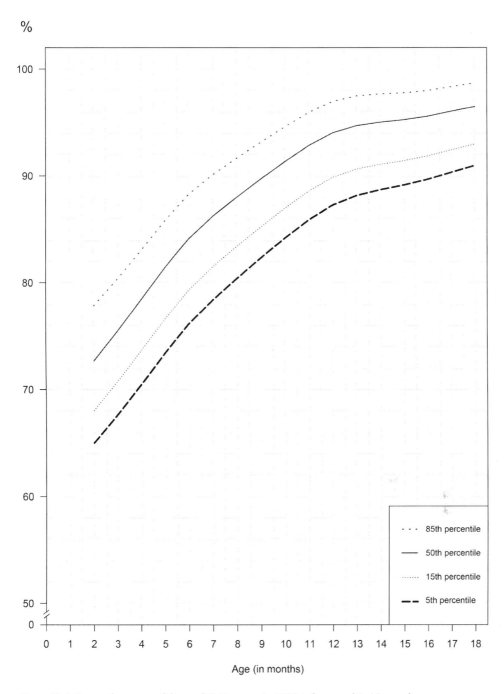

Figure 10.3 Percentile curves of the total IMP scores in 1700 infants aged 2–18 months

Table 10.4 Age–dependent percentile values of the total IMP scores

Age in months	P5	P15	P50	P85
3	68	71	75	80
4	70	74	78	83
5	73	77	81	86
6	76	79	84	88
7	78	81	86	90
8	80	83	88	92
9	82	85	90	93
10	84	87	91	95
11	86	89	93	97
12	87	90	94	97
13	88	91	95	98
14	89	91	95	98
15	89	91	95	98
16	90	92	96	98
17	90	92	96	98
18	91	93	96	99

P5=5th percentile, P15=15th percentile, P50=50th percentile, P85=85th percentile

Table 10.5 Percentile ranks of the total IMP score by age (in months)

Age	3	4	5	6	7	8	9	10	11	12	13	14	15	16	17	18
Score																
63	1															
64	1															
65	2															
66	3	1														
67	4	1														
68	6	2	1													
69	8	3	1													
70	12	4	1													
71	16	6	2	1												
72	22	9	3	1												
73	29	12	4	1	1											
74	37	17	6	2	1											
75	46	23	9	3	1	1										
76	55	29	12	5	2	1										
77	64	37	17	7	3	1										
78	71	46	23	10	4	2	1									
79	78	55	30	14	6	3	1									
80	83	64	37	18	9	4	2	1								
81	88	72	46	25	13	6	3	1								
82	91	79	55	32	18	9	4	2	1							
83	94	85	64	40	24	13	7	3	1	1						
84	95	89	73	49	31	18	10	5	2	1	1					

Age	3	4	5	6	7	8	9	10	11	12	13	14	15	16	17	18
85	97	93	80	58	39	25	14	7	3	2	1	1				
86	98	95	86	67	48	32	19	10	5	3	2	1	1			
87	99	97	91	76	58	41	26	15	8	4	3	2	1	1	1	
88	99	98	94	83	67	50	34	21	12	7	5	3	3	2	1	1
89	99	99	97	89	76	60	43	29	17	11	7	6	5	3	2	1
90		99	98	94	84	70	53	37	24	16	12	9	8	6	4	3
91			99	96	91	79	63	47	32	22	17	14	12	10	7	5
92				98	95	88	74	57	41	30	24	21	19	16	12	9
93				99	98	94	84	68	52	39	33	29	27	23	19	15
94					99	97	92	79	63	50	42	39	36	32	27	23
95						99	97	89	74	61	53	50	47	43	38	32
96							99	96	86	73	66	62	59	55	49	44
97								99	94	85	79	76	73	70	63	57
98									99	95	91	89	88	85	79	73
99										99	98	98	98	97	95	90
100											>99	>99	>99	>99	>99	>99

Table 10.6 IMP profile and suggestions for intervention

Domain	Suggestion for intervention
Variation	• Score ≥P15 (typical variation): high chance that therapeutic guidance results in beneficial effect • Score <P15 (atypical variation): inform families about the importance of variation: that is, of letting the infant experience motor activities in varied situations • Very limited repertoire: probably limited chances to improve repertoire. If the repertoire is repeatedly very limited, we suggest not to hesitate to use assistive devices: for example, adaptive seating systems, power mobility
Adaptability	• Score ≥P15 (typical adaptability): high chance that therapeutic guidance results in beneficial effect • Score <P15 (atypical adaptability): inform families that the infant's condition demands extra trial-and-error activities and opportunities; the infant will discover his own best strategies by trying out self-generated movements. Errors reflect a learning opportunity. Note that the strategies that the infant selects may differ from the strategies that typically developing infants select. We suggest accepting alternative strategies unless they are associated with a high risk of contractures and deformities.
Symmetry	• Score ≥P15 (typical symmetry): no specific suggestions for intervention • Score <P15 (asymmetry): inform families about the need to pay extra attention to the infant's more atypical side. Application of constrained induced movement therapy (baby-CIMT) and/or stimulation of bilateral upper extremity activities may be considered.
Fluency	For early intervention, this is the least important domain. Non-fluent movements are non-optimal but do not deserve specific attention during intervention.
Performance	The performance domain is an excellent tool to set goals for the next intervention period, as the domain describes step by step the sequences of infant motor development

Box 10.2 The two clinical examples in Chapter 1

Example 1: James

Wrap-up: at the age of three months, James was referred to a paediatric physiotherapist because of a positional head preference to the right side. The
IMP assessment at that age revealed that the variation and symmetry scores
were <P5, the performance score was <P15, and the fluency scores were
in the typical range. The therapist guides James and his family during the
following months. The intervention focuses on the implementation of
varying experiences of self-generated movements in daily caregiving activities. Special attention is given to play activities that challenge James to use
both hands. After three months, a follow-up IMP assessment is performed.
It shows that James has improved in the performance domain (P15–P50),
but his symmetry and variation scores continue to be low (<P5). Because
of the persistently low variation and symmetry scores, the therapist refers
the infant to a paediatric neurologist.

Continuation: two months later James, is diagnosed with a unilateral spastic
CP and referred to a paediatric rehabilitation centre. The therapist continues
early intervention and coaches the family on how to keep up with the
implementation of play activities that challenge James to use both arms
and hands in daily caregiving. For example, she provides suggestions on
toys that elicit bimanual activities. The IMP assessment at 12 months shows
that James's performance score follows the IMP percentile curves: his score
remains stable at P15–P50. The variation and symmetry scores improve
slightly but remain low (<P5). Importantly, these scores do not drop,
implying that deterioration of function by disuse has been prevented.
James's adaptability score was just at P15. This corresponds to the finding
that his performance scores follow a typical trajectory: James is really able
to learn from trial-and-error experiences.

Example 2: Janet

Wrap-up: a paediatrician was in charge of the follow-up of Janet, a girl born
very preterm. Janet had a complicated neonatal course, and the MRI scan
of her brain showed mild abnormalities. The paediatrician performs an
IMP assessment when Janet is eight months corrected age. She noticed
the following: (1) Janet has a re-assuring variation score (P15–P50), (2)
the symmetry and fluency scores are also within the typical range, and (3)
Janet's adaptability and performance scores are below the 15th percentile
(<P15). Janet's IMP profile suggests a relatively low risk of CP, but the
low scores on the adaptability and performance domain indicate that Janet
could profit from early intervention. This is prescribed.

Continuation: the therapist discusses the reasons for Janet's referral with the
caregivers. When she mentions that Janet presumably will profit from ample
varying experience of self-generated movements and being playfully challenged to try out new motor skills, the caregivers react hesitantly. They

say that Janet was so ill and so vulnerable in early life, they now wish to protect her from all further hardship. The therapist responds empathically, respectfully, and with understanding. She does not deny the caregivers' worries but provides them with suggestions on how to cope with these uncertainties. She also explains that infant development implies playing, exploring, having fun, and laughing about 'errors'. She mentions that adults actually can learn from the infants' relentless drive to explore and try out. The therapist and caregivers discuss a realistic goal for Janet to achieve in the next week. The caregivers suggest that they would like for Janet to learn to move around by herself. The IMP indicates that Janet is about to discover how to pivot when placed in the prone position. The therapist and caregivers discuss how they can integrate prone activities into daily life, including challenges to pivot. For example, they can do this during dressing on a play mattress on the floor.

When Janet is 12 months old, she revisits the paediatrician. Another IMP assessment is performed. It reveals that all Janet's IMP scores are in the typical range (P15–P50), including the adaptability and performance scores. The caregivers tell the paediatrician that not only has Janet profited from the early intervention, but they, as caregivers, have also. The intervention certainly helped them to get confidence in Janet's capacities and strengths.

Concluding remarks

The IMP is a reliable, valid, responsive, and norm-referenced assessment instrument for the evaluation of motor behaviour in at-risk infants up to the age of being able to walk independently for a couple of months. The IMP is an excellent tool to monitor the infant's motor developmental progress, and it furnishes concrete directions for early intervention (Table 10.6). In addition, low scores assist in the detection of infants with or at high risk of a developmental disorder.

References

Adams RJ, Courage ML (2002) Using a single test to measure human contrast sensitivity from early childhood to maturity. *Vision Research* 42: 1205–1210. doi: 10.1016/s0042-6989(02)00038-x.

Adolph KE, Hoch JE (2019) Motor development: embodied, embedded, enculturated and enabling. *Annual Review of Psychology* 70: 141–164. doi: 10.1146/annurev-psych-010418-102836.

Adolph KE, Vereijken B, Denny MA (1998) Learning to crawl. *Child Development* 69: 1299–1312. doi: 10.1111/j.1467-8624.1998.tb06213.x.

Aiello I, Rosati G, Sau GF, Patraskakis S, Bissakou M, Traccis S (1988) Tonic neck reflexes on upper limb flexor tone in man. *Experimental Neurology* 101: 41–49. doi: 10.1016/0014-4886(88) 90063-5.

Akhbari Ziegler S, Dirks T, Hadders-Algra M (2019) Coaching in early physical therapy intervention: the COPCA program as an example of translation of theory into practice. *Disability and Rehabilitation*41: 1846–1854. doi: 10.1080/09638288.2018.

Akhbari Ziegler S, von Rhein M, Meichtry A, et al. (2020) The coping with and caring for infants with special needs intervention was associated with improved motor development in preterm infants. *Acta Paediatrica*, epub ahead of print. doi: 10.1111/apa.15619.

Andrews K, Fitzgerald M (1994) The cutaneous withdrawal reflex in human neonates: sensitization, receptive fields, and the effect of contralateral stimulation. *Pain* 56: 95–101. doi: 10.1016/0304-3959(94)90154-6.

Ben-Ari Y, Spitzer NC (2010) Phenotypic checkpoints regulate neuronal development. *Trends in Neurosciences* 33: 485–492. doi: 10.1016/j.tins.2010.08.005.

Bonvicini C, Faraone SV, Scassellati C (2018) Common and specific genes and peripheral biomarkers in children and adults with attention-deficit/hyperactivity disorder. *World Journal of Biological Psychiatry* 19: 80–100. doi: 10.1080/15622975.2017.1282175.

Bornstein MH, Hahn CS, Suwalsky JT (2013) Physically developed and exploratory young infants contribute to their long-term academic achievement. *Psychological Science* 24: 1906–1917. doi: 10.1177/0956797613479974.

Bos AF, van Asperen RM, de Leeuw DM, Prechtl HF (1997) The influence of septicaemia on spontaneous motility in preterm infants. *Early Human Development* 50: 61–70. doi: 10.1016/s0378-3782(97)00093-5.

Bosanquet M, Copeland L, Ware R, Boyd R (2013) A systematic review of tests to predict cerebral palsy in young children. *Developmental Medicine and Child Neurology* 55: 418–426. doi: 10.1111/dmcn.12140.

Bottos M, Dalla Barba B, Stefani D, Pettenà G, Tonin C, D'Este A (1989) Locomotor strategies preceding independent walking: prospective study of neurological and language development in 424 cases. *Developmental Medicine and Child Neurology* 31: 25–34. doi: 10.1111/j.1469-8749.1989. tb08408.x.

Bouwstra H, Boersma ER, Boehm G, Dijck-Brouwer DA, Muskiet FA, Hadders-Algra M (2003) Exclusive breastfeeding of healthy term infants for at least 6 weeks improves neurological condition. *Journal of Nutrition* 133: 4243–4245. doi: 10.1093/jn/133.12.4243.

Boxum AG, La Bastide-Van Gemert S, Dijkstra LJ, Furda A, Reinders-Messelink HA, Hadders-Algra M (2019) Postural control during reaching while sitting and general motor behaviour when learning to walk. *Developmental Medicine and Child Neurology* 61: 555–562. doi: 10.1111/dmcn.13931.

Braddick O, Atkinson J (2011) Development of human visual function. *Vision Research* 51: 1588–1609. doi: 10.1016/j.visres.2011.02.018.

Braun K, Bock J, Wainstock T, et al. (2017) Experience-induced transgenerational (re)programming of neuronal structure and functions: impact of stress prior and during pregnancy. *Neuroscience and Biobehavioral Reviews* pii: S0149-7634(16)30731-X, epub only. doi: 10.1016/j.neubiorev.2017.05.021.

Bruijn SM, Massaad F, Maclellan MJ, Van Gestel L, Ivanenko YP, Duysens J (2013) Are effects of the symmetric and asymmetric tonic neck reflexes still visible in healthy adults? *Neuroscience Letters* 556: 89–92. doi: 10.1016/j.neulet.2013.10.028.

Burnett CN, Johnson EW (1971) Development of gait in childhood. II. *Developmental Medicine and Child Neurology* 13: 207–215. doi: 10.1111/j.1469-8749.1971.tb03246.x.

Burr DC, Morrone MC, Fiorentini A (1996) Spatial and temporal properties of infant colour vision. In: Vital-Durant F, Atkinson J, Braddick O, editors, *Infant Vision*. Oxford: Oxford University Press, pp. 63–78.

Cattaneo L, Pavesi G (2014) The facial motor system. *Neuroscience and Biobehavioral Reviews* 38: 135–159. https://doi.org/10.1016/j.neubiorev.2013.11.002.

Chamudot R, Parush S, Rigbi A, Horovitz R, Gross-Tsur V (2018) Effectiveness of modified constraint-induced movement therapy compared with bimanual therapy home programs for infants with hemiplegia: a randomized controlled trial. *American Journal of Occupational Therapy* 72: 7206205010p1–7206205010p9. doi: 10.5014/ajot.2018.025981.

Changeux J-P (1997) Variation and selection in neural function. *Trends in Neurosciences* 20: 291–293. doi: 10.1016/s0166-2236(97)88843-1.

Chervyakov AV, Sinitsyn DO, Piradov MA (2016) Variability of neuronal responses: types and functional significance in neuroplasticity and neural Darwinism. *Frontiers in Human Neuroscience* 10: 603. doi: 10.3389/fnhum.2016.00603.

De Graaf-Peters VB, Hadders-Algra M (2006) Ontogeny of the human central nervous system: what is happening when? *Early Human Development* 82: 257–266. doi: 10.1016/j.earlhumdev.2005.10.013.

de Vries AM, de Groot L (2002) Transient dystonias revisited: a comparative study of preterm and term children at 2 1/2 years of age. *Developmental Medicine and Child Neurology* 44: 415–421. doi: 10.1017/s0012162201002298.

de Vries JIP, Fong BF (2006) Normal fetal motility. An overview. *Ultrasound in Obstetrics and Gynecology* 27: 701–711. doi: 10.1002/uog.2740.

De Waal FBM (2003) Darwin's legacy and the study of primate visual communication. *Annals of the New York Academy of Sciences* 1000: 7–31. https://org.doi/10.1196/annals.1280.003.

Dirks T, Blauw-Hospers CH, Hulshof LJ, Hadders-Algra M (2011) Differences between the family-centered "COPCA" program and traditional infant physical therapy based on neurodevelopmental treatment principles *Physical Therapy* 91: 1303–1322. doi: 10.2522/ptj.20100207.

Dirks T, Hielkema T, Hamer EG, Reinders-Messelink HA, Hadders-Algra M (2016) Infant positioning in daily life may mediate associations between physiotherapy and child development – video-analysis of an early intervention RCT. *Research in Developmental Disabilities* 53–54: 147–157. doi: 10.1016/j.ridd.2016.02.006.

Drillien CM (1972) Abnormal neurologic signs in the first year of life in low-birthweight infants: possible prognostic significance. *Developmental Medicine and Child Neurology* 14: 575–584. doi: 10.1111/j.1469-8749.1972.tb02639.x.

Dubowitz LMS, Dubowitz V, Mercuri E (1999) *The neurological assessment of the preterm and full-term newborn infant*, 2nd edn. London: Mac Keith Press.

Edelman GM (1989) *Neural Darwinism: The theory of neuronal group selection*. Oxford: Oxford University Press.

Edelman GM (1993) Neural Darwinism: selection and reentrant signalling in higher brain function. *Neuron* 10: 115–125. doi: 10.1016/0896-6273(93)90304-a.

Einspieler C, Prechtl HFR, Bos AF, Ferrari F, Cioni G (2005) *Prechtl's method on the qualitative assessment of general movements in preterm, term and young infants.* London: Mac Keith Press.

Eliasson AC, Nordstrand L, Ek L, et al. (2018) The effectiveness of Baby-CIMT in infants younger than 12 months with clinical signs of unilateral cerebral palsy; an explorative study with randomized design. *Research in Developmental Disabilities* 72: 191–201. doi: 10.1016/j.ridd.2017.11.006.

Evans AL, Harrison LM, Stephens JA (1990) Maturation of the cutaneomuscular reflex recorded from the first dorsal interosseous muscle in man. *Journal of Physiology* 428: 425–440. doi: 10.1113/jphysiol.1990.sp018220.

Eyre JA (2007) Corticospinal tract development and its plasticity after perinatal injury. *Neuroscience and Biobehavioral Reviews* 31: 1136–1149. doi: 10.1016/j.neubiorev.2007.05.011.

Fabrizi L, Slater R, Worley A, et al. (2011) A shift in sensory processing that enables the developing human brain to discriminate touch from pain. *Current Biology* 21: 1552–1558. doi: 10.1016/j.cub.2011.08.010.

Festante F, Antonelli C, Chorna O, Corsi G, Guzzetta A (2019) Parent-infant interaction during the first year of life in infants at high risk for cerebral palsy: a systematic review of the literature. *Neural Plasticity* 2019: 5759694. doi: 10.1155/2019/5759694.

Forssberg H (1985) Ontogeny of human locomotor control. I. Infant stepping, supported locomotion and transition to independent locomotion.
Experimental Brain Research 57: 480–493. doi: 10.1007/BF00237835.

Gesell A, Amatruda CS (1947) *Developmental diagnosis: Normal and abnormal child development,* 2nd edn. New York: Harper & Row.

Greenough WT, Black JE, Wallace CS (1987) Experience and brain development. *Child Development* 58: 539–559. doi: 10.2307/1130197.

Groen SE, de Blécourt AC, Postema K, Hadders-Algra M (2005) General movements in early infancy predict neuromotor development at 9 to 12 years of age. *Developmental Medicine and Child Neurology* 47: 731–738. doi: 10.1017/S0012162205001544.

Growdon W, Ghika J, Henderson J, et al. (2000) Effects of proximal and distal muscles' groups contraction and mental stress on the amplitude and frequency of physiological finger tremor. An accelerometric study. *Electromyography and Clinical Neurophysiology* 40: 295–303.

Hadders-Algra M (2004) General movements: a window for early identification of children at high risk of developmental disorders. *Journal of Pediatrics* 145: S12–S18. doi: 10.1016/j.jpeds.2004.05.017.

Hadders-Algra M (2005) The neuromotor examination of the preschool child and its prognostic significance. *Mental Retardation and Developmental Disabilities Research Reviews* 11: 180–188. doi: 10.1002/mrdd.20069.

Hadders-Algra M (2008) Development of postural control. In: Hadders-Algra M, Brogren Carlberg E, editors, *Postural control: A key issue in developmental disorders.* London: Mac Keith Press, pp. 22–73.

Hadders-Algra M (2010) Variation and variability: key words in human motor development. *Physical Therapy* 90: 1823–1837. doi: 10.2522/ptj.20100006.

Hadders-Algra M (2018a) Early human brain development: starring the subplate. *Neuroscience and Biobehavioral Reviews* 92: 276–290. doi: 10.1016/j.neubiorev.2018.06.017.

Hadders-Algra M (2018b) Neural substrate and clinical significance of general movements: an update. *Developmental Medicine and Child Neurology* 60: 39–46. doi: 10.1111/dmcn.13540.

Hadders-Algra M (2018c) Early human motor development: from variation to the ability to vary and adapt. *Neuroscience and Biobehavioral Reviews* 90: 411–427. doi: 10.1016/j.neubiorev.2018.05.009.

Hadders-Algra M, editor (2021a) *Early detection and early intervention in developmental motor disorders – From neuroscience to participation in daily life.* London: Mac Keith Press, in press.

Hadders-Algra (2021b) Atypical motor development of the foetus and young infant. In: Hadders-Algra M, editor, *Early detection and early intervention in developmental motor disorders – From neuroscience to participation in daily life.* London: Mac Keith Press, in press.

Hadders-Algra (2021c) Early intervention in the first two years post-term. In: Hadders-Algra M, editor, *Early detection and early intervention in developmental motor disorders – From neuroscience to participation in daily life.* London: Mac Keith Press, in press.

Hadders-Algra (2021d) Early intervention in the neonatal period. In: Hadders-Algra M, editor, *Early detection and early intervention in developmental motor disorders – From neuroscience to participation in daily life*. London: Mac Keith Press, in press.

Hadders-Algra M, Boxum AG, Hielkema T, Hamer EG (2017) Effect of early intervention in infants at very high risk of cerebral palsy – a systematic review. *Developmental Medicine and Child Neurology* 59: 246–258. doi: 10.1111/dmcn.13331.

Hadders-Algra M, Brogren E, Forssberg H (1998) Postural adjustment during sitting at preschool age: presence of a transient toddling phase. *Developmental Medicine and Child Neurology* 40: 436–447. doi: 10.1111/j.1469-8749.1998.tb15393.x.

Hadders-Algra M, Brogren E, Katz-Salamon M, Forssberg H (1999) Periventricular leucomalacia and preterm birth have different detrimental effects on postural adjustments. *Brain* 122: 727–740. doi: 10.1093/brain/122.4.727.

Hadders-Algra M, Klip-Van den Nieuwendijk AWJ, Martijn A, Van Eykern LA (1997) Assessment of general movements: towards a better understanding of a sensitive method to evaluate brain function in young infants. *Developmental Medicine and Child Neurology* 39: 89–99. doi: 10.1111/j.1469-8749.1997.tb07390.x.

Hadders-Algra M, Tacke U, Pietz J, Rupp A, Philippi H (2019) Reliability and validity of the Standardized Infant NeuroDevelopmental Assessment Neurological Scale. *Developmental Medicine and Child Neurology* 61: 654–660. doi: 10.1111/dmcn.14045.

Hadders-Algra M, Tacke U, Pietz J, Rupp A, Philippi H (2020) Standardized Infant NeuroDevelopmental Assessment developmental and socio-emotional scales: reliability and predictive value in an at risk population. *Developmental Medicine and Child Neurology* 62: 845–853. doi: 10.1111/dmcn.14423.

Hakamada S, Hayakawa F, Kuno K, Tanaka R (1988) Development of the monosynaptic reflex pathway in the human spinal cord. *Brain Research* 470: 239–246. doi: 10.1016/0165-3806(88)90242-8.

Hamer EG, Bos AF, Hadders-Algra M (2011) Assessment of specific characteristics of abnormal general movements: does it enhance the prediction of cerebral palsy? *Developmental Medicine and Child Neurology* 53: 751–756. doi: 10.1111/j.1469-8749.2011.04007.x.

Hamer EG, Dijkstra LJ, Hooijsma SJ, Zijdewind I, Hadders-Algra M (2016) Knee jerk responses in infants at high risk for cerebral palsy: an observational EMG study. *Pediatric Research* 80: 363–370. doi: 10.1038/pr.2016.99.

Hartley C, Moultrie F, Gursul D, et al. (2016) Changing balance of spinal cord excitability and nociceptive brain activity in early human development. *Current Biology* 26: 1998–2002. doi: 10.1016/j.cub.2016.05.054.

Haynes RL, Borenstein NS, DesilvaTM, et al. (2005) Axonal development in the cerebral white matter of the human fetus and infant. *Journal of Comparative Neurology* 484: 156–167. doi: 10.1002/cne.20453.

Hecker E, Baer GD, Stark C, Herkenrath P, Hadders-Algra M (2016) Inter-and intra-rater reliability of the Infant Motor Profile in 3–18-month-old infants. *Pediatric Physical Therapy* 28: 217–222. doi: 10.1097/PEP.0000000000000244.

Heineman KR, Hadders-Algra M (2008) Evaluation of neuromotor function in infancy – a systematic review of available methods. *Journal of Developmental and Behavioral Pediatrics* 29: 315–323. doi: 10.1097/DBP.0b013e318182a4ea.

Heineman KR, Bos AF, Hadders-Algra M (2008) The Infant Motor Profile – a standardized and qualitative method to assess motor behaviour in infancy. *Developmental Medicine and Child Neurology* 50: 275–282. doi: 10.1111/j.1469-8749.2008.02035.x.

Heineman KR, Bos AF, Hadders-Algra M (2011) Infant Motor Profile and cerebral palsy – promising associations. *Developmental Medicine and Child Neurology* 53 (suppl 4): 40–45. doi: 10.1111/j.1469-8749.2011.04063.x.

Heineman KR, La Bastide-van Gemert S, Fidler V, Middelburg KJ, Bos AF, Hadders-Algra M (2010a) Construct validity of the Infant Motor Profile: relation with prenatal, perinatal and neonatal risk factors. *Developmental Medicine and Child Neurology* 52: e209–215. doi: 10.1111/j.1469-8749.2010.03667.x.

Heineman KR, Middelburg KJ, Bos AF, et al. (2013) Reliability and concurrent validity of the infant motor profile. *Developmental Medicine and Child Neurology* 55: 539–545. doi: 10.1111/dmcn.12100.

Heineman KR, Middelburg KJ, Hadders-Algra M (2010b) Development of adaptive motor behaviour in typically developing infants. *Acta Paediatrica* 99: 618–624. doi: 10.1111/j.1651-2227.2009. 01652.x.

Heineman KR, Schendelaar P, Van den Heuvel ER, Hadders-Algra M (2018) Motor development in infancy is related to cognitive function at 4 years of age. *Developmental Medicine and Child Neurology* 60: 1149–1155. doi: 10.1111/dmcn.13761.

Hempel MS (1993) Neurological development during toddling age in normal children and children at risk of developmental disorders. *Early Human Development* 34: 47–57. doi: 10.1016/0378-3782(93)90040-2.

Hepper PG, Shahidullah BS (1994) Development of fetal hearing. *Archives of Disease in Childhood* 71: F81–87.

Herlenius E, Lagercrantz H (2010) Neurotransmitters and neuromodulators. In: Lagercrantz H, Hanson MA, Ment LR, Peebles DM, editors, *The newborn brain: Neuroscience and clinical applications*, 2nd edn. Cambridge: Cambridge University Press, pp. 99–117.

Hernandez-Reif M, Field T, Diego M, Largie S (2001) Weight perception by newborns of depressed versus non-depressed mothers. *Infant Behavior and Development* 24: 305–316.

Hielkema T, Blauw-Hospers CH, Dirks T, Drijver-Messelink M, Bos AF, Hadders-Algra M (2011) Does physiotherapeutic intervention affect motor outcome in high-risk infants? An approach combining a randomized controlled trial and process evaluation. *Developmental Medicine and Child Neurology* 53: e8–15. doi: 10.1111/j.1469-8749.2010.03876.x.

Hielkema T, Hamer EG, Boxum AG, et al. (2020) LEARN2MOVE 0-2 years, a randomized early intervention trial for infants at very high risk of cerebral palsy: neuromotor, cognitive, and behavioural outcome. *Disability and Rehabilitation*, 42: 3752–3761. doi: 10.1080/09638288.2019.1610508.

Hoerder-Suabedissen A, Molnár Z (2015) Development, evolution and pathology of neocortical subplate neurons. *Nature Reviews Neuroscience* 16: 133–146, doi: 10.1038/nrn3915.

Hopkins B, Prechtl HFR (1984) A qualitative approach to the development of movements during early infancy. In: Prechtl HFR, editor, *Continuity of neural functions form prenatal to postnatal life*. Oxford: Blackwell Scientific Publication, pp. 179–197.

Huisman M, Koopman-Esseboom C, Lanting CI (1995) Neurological condition in 18-month-old children perinatally exposed to polychlorinated biphenyls and dioxins. *Early Human Development* 43: 165–176. doi: 10.1016/0378-3782(95)01674-0.

Issler H, Stephens JA. (1983) The maturation of cutaneous reflexes studied in the upper limb in man. *Journal of Physiology* 335: 643–654. doi: 10.1113/jphysiol.1983.sp014556.

Jeffery N, Spoor F (2004) Prenatal growth and development of the modern human labyrinth. *Journal of Anatomy* 204: 71–92. doi: 10.1111/j.1469-7580.2004.00250.x.

Johnson MH, Senju A, Tomalski P (2015) The two-process theory of face processing: modifications based on two decades of data from infants and adults. *Neuroscience and Biobehavioral Reviews* 50: 169–179. doi: 10.1016/j.neubiorev.2014.

Kang HJ, Kawasawa YI, Cheng F, et al. (2011) Spatio-temporal transcriptome of the human brain. *Nature* 478: 483–489. doi: 10.1038/nature10523.

Kikkert HK, Middelburg KJ, Hadders-Algra M (2010) Maternal anxiety is related to infant neurological condition, paternal anxiety is not. *Early Human Development* 86: 171–177. doi: 10.1016/j. earlhumdev.2010.02.004.

Kisilevsky BS, Hains SM, Lee K, et al. (2003) Effects of experience on fetal voice recognition. *Psychological Science* 14: 220–224. doi: 10.1111/1467-9280.02435.

Kolb B, Gibb R (2007) Brain plasticity and recovery from early cortical injury. *Developmental Psychobiology* 49: 107–118. doi: 10.1002/dev.20199.

Kostović I, Judas M (2010) The development of the subplate and thalamocortical connections in the human foetal brain. *Acta Paediatrica* 99: 1119–1127. doi: 10.1111/j.1651-2227.2010.01811.x.

Kostović I, Jovanov-Milošević N, Radoš M, et al. (2014a) Perinatal and early postnatal reorganization of the subplate and related cellular compartments in the human cerebral wall as revealed by histological and MRI approaches. *Brain Structure and Function* 219: 231–253. doi: 10.1007/s00429-012-0496-0.

Kostović I, Kostović-Srzentić M, Benjak V, Jovanov-Milošević N, Radoš M (2014b) Developmental dynamics of radial vulnerability in the cerebral compartments in preterm infants and neonates. *Frontiers in Neurology* 5: 139. doi: 10.3389/fneur.2014.00139.

Kostović I, Sedmak G, Vukšić M, Judaš M (2015) The relevance of human fetal subplate zone for developmental neuropathology of neuronal migration disorders and cortical dysplasia CNS. *CNS Neuroscience and Therapeutics* 21: 74–82. doi: 10.1111/cns.12333.

Krubitzer L, Kaas J (2005) The evolution of the neocortex in mammals: how is phenotypic diversity generated? *Current Opinion in Neurobiology* 15: 444–453. doi: 10.1016/j.conb.2005.07.003.

Kwon JY, Chang WH, Chang HJ, et al. (2014) Changes in diffusion tensor tractographic findings associated with constrained-induced movement therapy in young children with cerebral palsy. *Clinical Neurophysiology* 125: 2397–2403. doi: 10.1016/j.clinph.2014.02.025.

Lacquaniti F, Ivanenko YP, Zago M (2012) Development of human locomotion.
Current Opinion in Neurobiology 22: 822–828. doi: 10.1016/j.conb.2012.03.012.

Landry SH, Garner PW, Denson S, Swank PR, Baldwin C (1993) Low birth weight (LBW) infants' exploratory behavior at 12 and 24 months: effects of intraventricular hemorrhage and mothers' attention directing behaviors. *Research in Developmental Disabilities* 14: 237–249. doi: 10.1016/0891-4222(93)90033-g.

Largo RH, Molinari L, Weber M, Comenale Pinto L, Duc G (1985) Early development of locomotion: significance of prematurity, cerebral palsy and sex. *Developmental Medicine and Child Neurology* 27: 183–191. doi: 10.1111/j.1469-8749.1985.tb03768.x.

Lauffer H, Wenzel D (1986) Maturation of central somatosensory conduction time in infancy and childhood. *Neuropediatrics* 17: 72–74. doi: 10.1055/s-2008-1052504.

Ledebt A, Bril B (2000) Acquisition of upper body stability during walking in toddlers. *Developmental Psychobiology* 36: 311–324. doi: 10.1002/(sici)1098-2302(200005)36:4<311::aid-dev6>3.0.co;2-v.

Leighton AH, Lohmann C (2016) The wiring of developing sensory circuits – from patterned spontaneous activity to synaptic plasticity mechanisms. *Frontiers in Neural Circuits*10: 71. doi: 10.3389/fncir.2016.00071.

Leonard CT, Matsumoto T, Diedrich P (1995) Human myotatic reflex development of the lower extremities. *Early Human Development* 43: 75–93. doi: 10.1016/0378-3782(95)01669-t.

Lossi L, Merighi A (2003) In vivo cellular and molecular mechanisms of neuronal apoptosis in the mammalian CNS. *Progress in Neurobiology* 69: 287–312. doi: 10.1016/s0301-0082(03)00051-0.

Lüchinger AB, Hadders-Algra M, Van Kan CM, De Vries JIP (2008) Fetal onset of general movements. *Pediatric Research* 63: 191–195. doi: 10.1203/PDR.0b013e31815ed03e.

Lv J, Xin Y, Zhou W, Qiu Z (2013) The epigenetic switches for neural development and psychiatric disorders. *Journal of Genetics and Genomics* 40: 339–346. doi: 10.1016/j.jgg.2013.04.007.

Magnus R, de Kleijn A (1912) Die Abhängigkeit des Tonus der Extremitätenmusklen von der Kopfstellung. *Pflüger's Archiv, European Journal of Physiology* 145: 455–548.

Manning KY, Menon RS, Gorter JW, et al. (2016) Neuroplastic sensorimotor resting state network reorganization in children with hemiplegic cerebral palsy treated with constraint-induced movement therapy. *Journal of Child Neurology* 31: 220–226. doi: 10.1177/0883073815588995.

Martakis K, Hünseler C, Herkenrath P, Thangavelu K, Kribs A, Roth B (2017) The flexion withdrawal reflex increases in premature infants at 22–26 weeks of gestation due to changes in spinal cord excitability. *Acta Paediatrica* 106: 1079–1084. doi: 10.1111/apa.13854.

Mattock K, Amitay S, Moore DR (2012) Auditory development and learning. In: Plack CJ, editor, *Oxford Handbook of Auditory Science: Hearing*. Oxford: Oxford On-line Handbooks. doi: 10.1093/oxfordhb/9780199233557.013.0013.

McDonough SM, Clowry GJ, Miller S, Eyre JA (2001) Reciprocal and Renshaw (recurrent) inhibition are functional in man at birth. *Brain Research* 899: 66–81. doi: 10.1016/s0006-8993(01)02151-5.

McGraw MB (1943) *The neuromuscular maturation of the human infant*. Reprinted in 1989: *Classics in Developmental Medicine*, no. 4. London: Mac Keith Press.

McInerney MS, Reddihough DS, Carding PN, Swanton R, Walton CM, Imms C (2019) Behavioural interventions to treat drooling in children with neurodisability: a systematic review. *Developmental Medicine and Child Neurology* 61: 39–48. doi: 10.1111/dmcn.14048.

Meltzoff AN, Kuhl PK, Movellan J, Sejnowski TJ (2009) Foundations for a new science of learning. *Science* 325: 284–288. doi: 10.1126/science.1175626.

Mercer ME, Drodge SC, Courage ML, Adams RJ. (2014) A pseudoisochromatic test of color vision for human infants. *Vision Research* 100: 72–77. doi: 10.1016/j.visres.2014.04.006.

Miranda SB (1970) Visual abilities and pattern preferences of premature infants and full-term neonates. *Journal of Experimental Child Psychology* 10: 189–205. doi: 10.1016/0022-0965(70)90071-8.

Molina M, Jouen F (2003) Haptic intramodal comparison of texture in human neonates. *Developmental Psychobiology* 42: 378–385. doi: 10.1002/dev.10111.

Moon C, Lagercrantz H, Kuhl PK (2013) Language experienced in utero affects vowel perception after birth: a two-country study. *Acta Paediatrica* 102: 156–160. doi: 10.1111/apa.12098.

Morgan C, Darrah J, Gordon AM, et al. (2016) Effectiveness of motor interventions in infants with cerebral palsy: a systematic review. *Developmental Medicine and Child Neurology* 58: 900–909. doi: 10.1111/dmcn.13105.

Norcia AM, Gerhard HE (2015) Development of three-dimensional perception in human infants. *Annual Review of Vision Science* 1: 569–594. doi: 10.1146/annurev-vision-082114-035835.

Novak I, Morgan C, Adde L, et al. (2017) Cerebral Palsy: advances in early diagnosis. *Journal of the American Medical Association Pediatrics* 171: 897–907. doi: 10.1001/jamapediatrics.2017.1689.

Novak I, Morgan C, Fahey M, et al. (2020) State of the evidence traffic lights 2019: systematic review of interventions for preventing and treating children with cerebral palsy. *Current Neurology and Neuroscience Reports* 20: 3. doi: 10.1007/s11910-020-1022-z.

Ortega JA, Memi F, Radonjic N, et al. (2018) The subventricular zone: a key player in human neocortical development. *Neuroscientist* 24: 156–170. doi: 10.1177/1073858417691009.

O'Sullivan MC, Eyre JA, Miller S (1991) Radiation of phasic stretch reflex in biceps brachii to muscles of the arm in man and its restriction during development. *Journal of Physiology* 439: 529–543.

Peiper A (1963) *Cerebral function in infancy and childhood*, 3rd edn. New York: Consultants Bureau.

Petanjek Z, Judaš M, Šimic G, et al. (2011) Extraordinary neoteny of synaptic spines in the human prefrontal cortex. *Proceedings of the National Academy of Sciences of the United States of America* 108: 13281–13286. doi: 10.1073/pnas.1105108108.

Piña-Garza EJ, James KC (2019) *Fenichel's clinical pediatric neurology: A signs and symptoms approach*, 8th edn. Amsterdam: Elsevier.

Piper MC, Darrah J (1994) *Motor assessment of the developing infant*. Philadelphia, PA: W.B. Saunders Company.

Prado MTA, Fernani DCGL, Silva TDD, Smorenburg ARP, Abreu LC, Monteiro CBM (2017) Motor learning paradigm and contextual interference in manual computer tasks in individuals with cerebral palsy. *Research in Developmental Disabilities* 64: 56–63. doi: 10.1016/j.ridd.2017.03.006.

Prechtl HFR (1977) *The neurological examination of the full term newborn*, 2nd edn. London: Heinemann Medical Books.

Prechtl HR (1990) Qualitative changes of spontaneous movements in fetus and preterm infant are a marker of neurological dysfunction. *Early Human Development* 23: 151–158. doi: 10.1016/0378-3782(90)90011-7.

R Core Team (2019) R: A language and environment for statistical computing. R Foundation for Statistical Computing, Vienna, Austria. https://www.R-project.org/

Raichle ME (2015) The restless brain: how intrinsic activity organizes brain function. *Philosophical Transactions of the Royal Society of London. Series B, Biological Sciences* 370: 20140172. doi: 10.1098/rstb.2014.0172.

Ricci D, Romeo DM, Serrao F, et al. (2010) Early assessment of visual function in preterm infants: how early is early? *Early Human Development* 86: 29–33. doi: 10.1016/j.earlhumdev.2009.11.004.

Rigby RA, Stasinopoulos DM (2005) Generalized additive models for location, scale and shape, (with discussion). *Journal of the Royal Statistical Society, Series C (Applied Statistics)* 54: 507–554. doi: 10.1111/j.1467-9876.2005.00510.x.

Robson P (1970) Shuffling, hitching, scooting or sliding: some observations in 40 otherwise normal children. *Developmental Medicine and Child Neurology* 2: 608–617. doi: 10.1111/j.1469-8749.1970.tb01970.x.

Rochat P (1987) Mouthing and grasping in neonates: evidence for the early detection of what hard or soft substances afford for action. *Infant Behavior and Development* 10: 435–449.

Ruff HF (1984) Infants' manipulative exploration of objects: effects of age and object characteristics. *Developmental Psychology* 20: 9–20.

Sakzewski L, Sicola E, Verhage CH, Sgandurra G, Eliasson AC (2019) Development of hand function during the first year of life in children with unilateral cerebral palsy. *Developmental Medicine and Child Neurology* 61: 563–569. doi: 10.1111/dmcn.14091.

Sargent B (2021) Psychometric properties of standardized tests. In: Hadders-Algra M, editor, *Early detection and early intervention in developmental motor disorders – From neuroscience to participation in daily life*. London: Mac Keith Press, in press.

Sarnat HB (2004) Ontogenesis of striate muscle. In: RA Polin, WW Fox and SH Abman, editors, *Fetal and neonatal physiology*, Vol. 2, 3rd edn. Philadelphia: Saunders, pp 1849–1870.

Sgandurra G, Bartalena L, Cecchi F, et al. (2016) A pilot study on early home-based intervention through an intelligent baby gym (CareToy) in preterm infants. *Research in Developmental Disabilities*53–54: 32–42. doi: 10.1016/j.ridd.2016.01.013.

Sgandurra G, Lorentzen J, Inguaggiato E, et al. (2017) A randomized clinical trial in preterm infants on the effects of a home-based early intervention with the CareToy System. *PLoS One* 12: e0173521. doi: 10.1371/journal.pone.0173521.

Sherrington CS (1906) *The integrative action of the nervous system*. London: Constable.

Smith LB, Thelen E (2003) Development as a dynamic system. *Trends in Cognitive Sciences* 7: 343–348. doi: 10.1016/s1364-6613(03)00156-6.

Spencer JP, Perone S, Buss AT (2011) Twenty years and going strong: a dynamic systems revolution in motor and cognitive development. *Child Development Perspectives* 5: 260–266. doi: 10.1111/j.1750-8606.2011.00194.x.

Spittle A, Orton J, Anderson PJ, Boyd R, Doyle LW (2015) Early developmental intervention programmes provided post hospital discharge to prevent motor and cognitive impairment in preterm infants. *Cochrane Database of Systematic Reviews* 11: CD005495. doi: 10.1002/14651858.CD005495.pub4.

Straathof EJM, Heineman KR, Hamer EG, Hadders-Algra M (2020) Prevailing head position to one side in early infancy – a population-based study. *Acta Paediatrica* 109: 1423–1429. doi: 10.1111/apa.15112.

Sterling C, Taub E, Davis D, et al. (2013) Structural neuroplastic change after constraint-induced movement therapy in children with cerebral palsy. *Pediatrics* 131: e1664–1669. doi: 10.1542/peds.2012-2051.

Streri A, Gentaz E (2003) Cross-modal recognition of shape from hand to eyes in human newborns. *Somatosensory and Motor Research* 20: 13–18.

Takahashi H, Yokota R, Kanzaki R (2013) Response variance in functional maps: neuronal Darwinism revisited. *PLoS One* 8: e68705. doi: 10.1371/journal.pone.0068705.

Teulier C, Ulrich BD, Martin B (2011) Functioning of peripheral Ia pathways in infants with typical development: responses in antagonistic muscle pairs. *Experimental Brain Research* 208: 581–593. doi: 10.1007/s00221-010-2506-x.

Thelen E (1995) Motor development. A new synthesis. *American Psychologist* 50: 79–95. doi: 10.1037//0003-066x.50.2.79.

Thunberg G, Livingstone R, Buchholz M, Field D (2021) Environmental adaptations. In: Hadders-Algra M, editor, *Early detection and early intervention in developmental motor disorders – From neuroscience to participation in daily life*. London: Mac Keith Press, in press.

Touwen BCL (1976) *Neurological development in infancy*. London: Heinemann Medical Books.

Touwen BC, Hadders-Algra M (1983) Hyperextension of neck and trunk and shoulder retraction in infancy – a prognostic study. *Neuropediatrics* 14: 202–205. doi: 10.1055/s-2008-1059579.

Trevarthen C (1984) How control of movements develops. In: Whiting HTA, editor, *Human motor actions: Bernstein reassessed.* Amsterdam: Elsevier, pp. 223–261.

Tveten KM, Hadders-Algra M, Strand LI, Van Iersel PAM, Rieber J, Dragesund T (2020) Intra- and Inter-Rater Reliability of the Infant Motor Profile in Infants in Primary Health Care. *Physical and Occupational Therapy in Pediatrics* 31: 1–11. doi: 10.1080/01942638.2020.1720331.

van der Heide JC, Fock JM, Otten B, Stremmelaar E, Hadders-Algra M (2005) Kinematic characteristics of postural control during reaching in preterm children with cerebral palsy. *Pediatric Research* 58: 586–593. doi: 10.1203/01.pdr.0000176834.47305.26.

Vitrac C, Benoit-Marand M (2017) Monoaminergic modulation of motor cortex function. *Frontiers in Neural Circuits* 11: 72. doi: 10.3389/fncir.2017.00072.

Volpe JJ (2009a) Brain injury in premature infants: a complex amalgam of destructive and developmental disturbances. *Lancet Neurology* 8: 110–124. doi: 10.1016/S1474-4422(08)70294-1.

Volpe JJ (2009b) Cerebellum of the premature infant: rapidly developing, vulnerable, clinically important. *Journal of Child Neurology* 24: 1085–1104. doi: 10.1177/0883073809338067.

Weissman BM, DiScenna AO, Leigh RJ (1989) Maturation of the vestibulo-ocular reflex in normal infants during the first 2 months of life. *Neurology* 39: 534–538. doi: 10.1212/wnl.39.4.534.

Wiener-Vacher SR, Wiener SI (2017) Video head impulse test with a remote camera system: normative values of semicircular canal vestibulo-ocular reflex gain in infants and children. *Frontiers in Neurology* 8: 434. doi: 10.3389/fneur.2017.00434.

Wilson PH, Smits-Engelsman B, Caeyenberghs K, et al. (2017) Cognitive and neuroimaging findings in developmental coordination disorder: new insights from a systematic review of recent research. *Developmental Medicine and Child Neurology* 59: 1117–1129. doi: 10.1111/dmcn.13530.

Wu YC, Bouwstra H, Heineman K, Hadders-Algra M (2020a) Atypical general movements in the general population: prevalence over the last 15 years and associated factors. *Acta Paediatrica*, 109: 2762–2769. doi: 10.1111/apa.15329.

Wu Y-C, Heineman KR, la Bastide-van Gemert S, Kuiper D, Drenth Olivares M, Hadders-Algra M (2020b) Motor behaviour in infancy is associated with cognitive, neurological and behavioural function in 9-year-old children born to parents with reduced fertility. *Developmental Medicine and Child Neurology*, 62: 1089–1095. doi: 10.1111/dmcn.14520.

Wu YC, van Rijssen IM, Buurman MT, Dijkstra LJ, Hamer EG, Hadders-Algra M (2020c) Temporal and spatial localization of general movement complexity and variation – why Gestalt assessment requires experience. *Acta Paediatrica*, epub ahead of print. doi: 10.1111/apa.15300.

Yakovlev PL, Lecours AR (1967) The myelogenetic cycles of regional maturation of the brain. In: Minkowski A, editor, *Regional development of the brain in early life.* Oxford: Blackwell, pp. 3–70.

Young YH (2015) Assessment of functional development of the otolithic system in growing children: a review. *International Journal of Pediatric Otorhinolaryngology* 79: 435–442. doi: 10.1016/j.ijporl.2015.01.015.

Index

Note: Page numbers in *italics* indicate a figure and page numbers in **bold** indicate a table on the corresponding page.

abdominal crawling *66*, 66–67
adaptability 13, 14; domain score 18, 19; of facial expression 129
adaptability domain of IMP 18, 134–137, *135*, **136**, **143**
adaptability of movements while prone: crawling 70–71, *71*; of head 59–60, *60*
adaptability of movements while supine 31; of hands while reaching, grasping, and manipulating 52; of head 33–34, *34*; reaching of arms 46, 50–51, *51*
adaptability of reaching while sitting: of hand movements while reaching, grasping, and manipulating 124–125, *125*; reaching movements of arms 120–121, *121*
adaptability of sitting position: ability of movement 83–84, *84*; getting into sitting position 87–88, *88*
adaptability while standing and walking: of arm and hand movements 104, *105*; of foot movements 111–112, *112*; of leg movements 108–109, *109*; of standing up behaviour 96, *97*; of trunk movements 106, *107*
Alberta Infant Motor Scale (AIMS) 25
arm movement adaptability: reaching while sitting 120–121, *121*; reaching while supine 46, 50–51, *51*
arm movement variation: reaching while sitting 119, *120*; reaching while supine 46, 49, *50*; while supine 39, *39*
arm posture and movements while walking 100–102, *101*, *102*
arms and hands movements, reaching, grasping, and manipulation of objects while sitting, asymmetry of 118–119
arms and hands movements, while walking independently: adaptability of 104, *105*; variation in 103
arms and hands while prone: functional ability 63–64, *64*; posture and movements during activity, asymmetry 65

arms, voluntary use in sitting position *81*, 81
assessment procedures of motor behaviour 19, **20–21**
asymmetrical tonic neck reflex (ATNR) 36, *36*
asymmetry, symmetry domain of IMP 18, **134**, 137, **143**
asymmetry of arms and hands movements, in reaching, grasping, and manipulation of objects while sitting 118–119
asymmetry of sitting position: of head position *75*, 75–76; of trunk and legs posture 79–80; of upper extremities 80
asymmetry while prone: arms and hands movements during activity 65; of head position 58, *58*, *59*
asymmetry while supine: of head position 34–35, *35*; reaching, grasping, and manipulating objects 48–49
asymmetry while walking independently: leg posture and movements 107; upper extremities, posture and movements 102–103
auditory system, development of 10–11
axon elimination 7

balance while walking independently 99–100, *100*
balancing capacities 99
bear crawling 66, *66*
behavioural state of infant 21
bottom shuffling 89, *89*
brain development 4–8, *5*
brain lesions 14, 134
bunny hopping 66

CareToy system 27
cerebellum 7
cerebral palsy (CP) 1, 25, 27, 133–134, 137, 138, 140
clinical application 19–23, 132–145; assessment form 22, *23*; assessment typical course 19; behavioural state and movement quantity 21; examples of 2, 144–145; IMP percentile curves

132–133, *135, 139, 141*; motor domains *see* motor domains of IMP; recommendations on practical procedures **20–21**; requirements 21–22; total IMP score 140, *141*, **142–143**
concurrent validity 24, 25, **26**
construct validity 24, 25
Coping with and Caring for Infants with Special Needs (COPCA) 27, 137
cortical plate 5, *6*
cortical subplate 4–6, *6, 7*, 16
crawling movement while prone: adaptability of 70–71, *71*; pre-crawling movements of legs, variation in 67–68; progression, development of crawling 65–67, *66*; variation in 69–70
cutaneous information, development of processing of 9–10

developmental coordination disorder (DCD) 1, 136
developmental disorders 1, 133–134, 136, 138, 140
discriminative measurement/instrument 2, 17
drooling *129*, 129–130
Dynamic Systems Theory 11

Edelman, Gerald 1
en bloc 70, 87, 105
environment 11, 137, 138
evaluative measurement/instrument 2, 17
examples of clinical application 2, 144–145

facial expression: adaptability of 129; variation in 128
finger movement variation while supine *39*, 40
fingers and hands, manipulative behaviour while supine 37–38, *38*
fluency: of motor behaviour 130–131; of motor behaviour while supine 53; of movements during prereaching and reaching 126–127; of movements while walking independently 113
fluency domain of IMP 18, **134**, 137–138, **143**
foot movements while walking independently: adaptability of 111–112, *112*; variation in 111

gender-neutral intentions 3
General Movement Assessment 1, 3
general movements 1, 15
genes/genetics 11–13
getting into sitting position *85*, 85–86, *86*; adaptability of 87–88, *88*; variation in 87
glial cells 6
grasping types 121–123, *123*
grasping while sitting *see* reaching, grasping, and manipulation of objects while sitting
grasping while supine: adaptability of hand movements 52; assessment procedures **21**, 30, *31*, 45; of objects 46–47, *48*; of objects,

presence of asymmetry 48–49; variation in hand movements 51–52
gustatory information, development of processing of 11

half sitting position 85, *86*
hand movements, while reaching, grasping, and manipulating: adaptability of, while sitting 124–125, *125*; adaptability of, while supine 52; variation in, while sitting 124; variation in, while supine 51–52
hands and arms while prone: functional ability 63–64, *64*; posture and movements during activity, asymmetry 65
hands and fingers, manipulative behaviour while supine 37–38, *38*
head movement in sitting position, control of 72, 73–75, *74*
head movement while prone: adaptability 59–60, *60*; lift 56, *57*, 58, *58*; variation *57*, 59
head movement while supine: adaptability of 33–34, *34*; control of 29, 32, *32*; variation in 33
head position, asymmetry, prevailing to one side 137; in sitting position *75*, 75–76; while prone 58, *58, 59*; while supine 34–35, *35*
heel-toe gait 109–110, *110*
high guard posture 100–104, *101*
hyperextension of neck and trunk while supine 37, *37*

IMP-SINDA project 24, 25, **26**, 133
Infant Motor Profile (IMP) 1–3; design of 17–19; implementation in clinical practice 19–23, 132–145 (*see also* clinical application); intervention suggestions **143** (*see also* intervention); motor domains of 17–18, 44, 133–140 (*see also* motor domains of IMP); percentile curves 132–133, *135, 139, 141*; psychometric properties of 24–27; scores 18–19, *23*, 140, *141*, **142–143**
inferior pincer grasp 121, 122, *123*, 124
intelligence quotient (IQ) 27, 136, 138, 140
inter-rater reliability 24, 25
intervention 27, 134, 136–138, 140, **143**
intra-rater reliability 24, 25
items observed throughout assessment 128–131; drooling *129*, 129–130; facial expression, adaptability of 129; facial expression, variation in 128, *128*; motor behaviour fluency 130–131; stereotyped tongue protrusion 130; tremor 130

jerky movements 53, 113, 127, 131, 138

leg movement adaptability, while walking independently 108–109, *109*

leg movement variation: pre-crawling movements while prone 67–68; while supine 42, *43*; while walking independently 108
leg posture, asymmetry: and movements while walking independently 107; while sitting 79–80
lesions of brain 14, 134
locomotion 54
long-leg sitting 73
lordosis 78, 105
Lorenz, Konrad 3

manipulation while sitting *see* reaching, grasping, and manipulation of objects while sitting
manipulation while supine: adaptability of hand movements 52; assessment procedures **21**, 30, *31*, 45; of fingers and hands 37–38, *38*; of objects 46–47, *48*; of objects, presence of asymmetry 48–49; variation in hand movements 51–52
milestones 13, 138
monoaminergic systems 14, 136
motor development 14–16; atypical, and NGST 13–14; typical, and NGST 11–13, *12*
motor domains of IMP 17–18, 133–140, **143**; adaptability domain 18, 134–137, *135*, **136**; fluency domain 18, **134**, 137–138; performance domain 18, 138–140, *139*, **140**; symmetry domain 18, **134**, 137; variation domain 17, 133–134, **134**
motor skills 15, 138
movement quantity 21
muscle development 8
myelination 6–7

neck and trunk, hyperextension while supine 37, *37*
neural development 4–8
Neural Maturationist Theories 11
neurodevelopmental assessment 1
Neuronal Group Selection Theory (NGST) 1, 11; and atypical motor development 13–14; and typical motor development 11–13, *12*
neurotransmitters 7
noli me tangere 90
norm data **24**; *see also* percentile curves

olfactory information, development of processing of 11

palmar grasp 122, *123*
pelvis tilting while supine 40–42, *41*, *42*
percentile curves 132–133, *135*, *139*, *141*
performance domain of IMP 18, 138–140, *139*, **140**, **143**
permissions 3
pincer grasp 121, 122, *123*, 124

pivoting 65–67
postural control 15
Prechtl, Heinz 3
pre-crawling movements, variation in 67–68
prediction of developmental outcome 3
predictive validity 24, 25, 27
prereaching movements 46–47, 51, 116–117, 126–127
preterm birth 3, 8–9, 14, 24, 133–134, 136
primary variability *12*, 12–13, 14
prone, motor behaviour assessment 54–71; arms and hands functional ability 63–64, *64*; arms and hands movements during activity, asymmetry 65; assessment procedures **20**, 54–56, *55*; crawling adaptability 70–71, *71*; crawling, progression 65–67, *66*; crawling variation 69–70; head lift 56, *57*, 58, *58*; head movement adaptability 59–60, *60*; head movement variation *57*, 59; head position, asymmetry 58, *58*, *59*; legs, variation in pre-crawling movements 67–68; rolling from prone into supine 68–69, *69*; shoulder girdle functional ability 61–63, *62*
propioception, development of 9
psychometric properties of IMP 24–27
pull-to-sit 72

radial palmar grasp 122, *123*
reaching, grasping, and manipulation of objects while sitting 114–127; ability to reach, grasp, and manipulate objects 116–117, *117*, *118*; arm and hand movements, asymmetry of 118–119; arms, reaching movements, adaptability of 120–121, *121*; arms, reaching movements, variation in 119, *120*; assessment procedures **21**, 114–116, *115*; fluency of movements during prereaching and reaching 126–127; grasping type 121–123, *123*; hand movements, adaptability of 124–125, *125*; hand movements, variation in 124; tremor during prereaching and reaching 126
reaching while supine: adaptability of arm movements 50–51, *51*; adaptability of hand movements 52; assessment procedures **21**, 30, *31*, 45; of objects 46–47, *48*; of objects, presence of asymmetry 48–49; tremor during 52–53; variation in arm movements 46, 49, *50*; variation in hand movements 51–52
recommendations for assessment 21–22, *22*
reduced repertoire 14
reliability of IMP 24, 25
responsiveness to change of IMP 27
rolling: from prone into supine 68–69, *69*; from supine into prone 31, 44–45, *45*

sacral sitting 78
scissor grasp 122

scores, IMP: calculation of 18–19; score form
    for supine position *23*; total score 140, *141*,
    142–143
secondary variability *12*, 13, 14
selection, adaptive 13–14, 18
semi-high guard 100–104
sensory systems, development of 8–11, 13
shoulder girdle, functional ability while prone
    61–63, *62*
SINDA (Standardized Infant
    NeuroDevelopmental Assessment) 24, 25, **26**
sitting position, motor behaviour assessment
    72–89; arms, voluntary use of *81*, 81;
    assessment procedures **20**, 72–73; bottom
    shuffling 89, *89*; getting into sitting position
    85, 85–86, *86*; getting into sitting position,
    adaptability of 87–88, *88*; getting into sitting
    position, variation in 87; head movement
    control 72, 73–75, *74*; head position,
    asymmetry *75*, 75–76; sitting ability 76–77,
    77; sitting movements, adaptability of 83–84,
    84; sitting movements, variation in 82, 82,
    83; trunk and legs posture, asymmetry 79–80;
    trunk posture while sitting independently *78*,
    78–79, *79*; upper extremities, asymmetry 80
sluggish movements 53, 113, 127, 131
Standardized Infant NeuroDevelopmental
    Assessment *see* SINDA
standing, motor behaviour assessment 90–113;
    ability to stand 91–93, *92*; assessment
    procedures **20**, 90–91; standing up 93–94, *94*;
    standing up behaviour, adaptability of 96, *97*;
    standing up behaviour, variation in 95, *95*;
    trunk movements, adaptability of 106, *107*;
    trunk movements, variation in 105–106
stereotyped tongue protrusion 130
stereotypy (or stereotyped movements) 52, 65,
    103, 108, 124
stiff movements 53, 113, 127, 131, 138
stress during early life 14, 136
supine, motor behaviour assessment 28–53; arm
    movement variation 38, *39*; arms, adaptability
    of reaching movements 46, 50–51, *51*; arms,
    variation in reaching movements 46, 49, *50*;
    assessment procedures **20**, 28–31, *29*, *45*;
    finger movement variation *39*, 40; fluency
    of motor behaviour 53; hand movements,
    adaptability while reaching, grasping, and
    manipulating 52; hand movements, variation
    while reaching, grasping, and manipulating
    51–52; hands and fingers, manipulative
    behaviour 37–38, *38*; head movement
    adaptability 33–34, *34*; head movement
    control 29, 32, *32*; head movement variation
    32; head position asymmetry 34–35, *35*;
    IMP-score form *23*; leg movement variation
    42, *43*; pelvis tilting 40–42, *41*, *42*; posture,

presence of ATNR 36, *36*; posture, presence
    of hyperextension of neck and trunk 37,
    37; reaching, grasping, and manipulating
    objects 46–47, *48*; reaching, grasping, and
    manipulating objects, asymmetry in 48–49;
    rolling from supine into prone 44–45, *45*; toe
    movement variation *43*, 44; tremor during
    prereaching and reaching 52–53
symmetry domain of IMP 18, **134**, 137, **143**;
    see also asymmetry entries

toddling behaviour 106
toe movement variation while supine *43*, 44
tongue protrusion, stereotyped 130
Touwen infant neurological examination 25
toys, recommended for assessment 22, *22*,
    114–115
transient dystonia 37
tremors 52–53, 126, 130
trial and error 13–15, 136
trunk: hyperextension of neck and trunk
    while supine 37, *37*; posture while sitting,
    asymmetry 79–80; posture while sitting
    independently *78*, 78–79, *79*
trunk movements, while standing and walking:
    adaptability of 106, *107*; variation in 105–106

upper extremities posture and movements of,
    asymmetry: in sitting position 80; while
    walking 102–103

validity of IMP 24, 25–27
variability 16n1; primary *12*, 12–13, 14;
    secondary *12*, 13, 14
variation 1, 16n1; in facial expression 128
variation domain of IMP 17, 133–134, **134**, **143**
variation in movements while prone: of crawling
    69–70; of head *57*, 59; of pre-crawling 67–68
variation in movements while supine 31; of arms
    38, *39*; arms, reaching of 46, 49, *50*; of fingers
    39, 40; of hands while reaching, grasping, and
    manipulating 51–52; of head 33; of legs 42,
    43; of toes *43*, 44
variation in reaching while sitting: of hand
    movements while reaching, grasping, and
    manipulating 124; reaching movements of
    arms 119, *120*
variation in sitting movements *82*, 82, *83*; in
    getting into sitting position 87
variation while standing and walking: in arm and
    hand movements 103; in foot movements 111;
    in leg movements 108; in standing up behaviour
    95, *95*; in trunk movements 105–106
vestibular system, development of 9
video camera 21–22
visual attention 31, 114
visual system, development of 8

walking, motor behaviour assessment 90–113; ability to walk 96–97, *98*; arm and hand movements, adaptability of 104, *105*; arm and hand movements, variation in 103; arm posture and movements 100–102, *101*, *102*; assessment procedures **20–21**, 90–91; balance while walking independently 99–100, *100*; fluency of movements 113; foot movements, adaptability of 111–112, *112*; foot movements, variation in 111; heel-toe gait 109–110, *110*; leg movements, adaptability of 108–109, *109*; leg movements, variation in 108; leg posture and movements, asymmetry in 107; trunk movements, adaptability of 106, *107*; trunk movements, variation in 105–106; upper extremities, posture and movements, asymmetry 102–103

website 18, 22, 27

W sitting 73

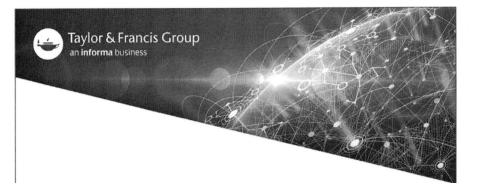

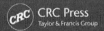

Printed in the United States
By Bookmasters